National Health Education Standards

SECOND EDITION

ACHIEVING EXCELLENCE

National Health Education Standards

SECOND EDITION

ACHIEVING EXCELLENCE

Developed by the
Joint Committee on
National Health Education Standards

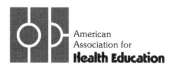

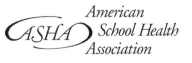

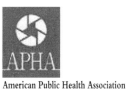

American Public Health Association

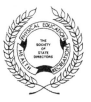

 Sponsored by the American Cancer Society

Cover Design: Marty Benoit
Text Design/Composition: Graphic Composition, Inc., Athens, Georgia.
Printed and bound in Canada.

ISBN: 978-0-944235-73-7

Library of Congress Cataloging-in-Publication Data

Joint Committee on National Health Education Standards.
  National health education standards : achieving excellence /
  developed by the Joint Committee on National Health Education Standards.—2nd ed.
    p.   cm.
  ISBN-13: 978-0-944235-73-7
  ISBN-10: 0-944235-73-5
  1. Health education—Standards—United States. I. Title.
RA440.3.U5J65 2007
613.071—dc22

                              2006037881

Some of the illustrations in this text (Figures 4.3 and 4.5) were provided by the Association for Supervision and Curriculum Development (ASCD). ASCD is a worldwide community of educators advocating sound policies and sharing best practices to achieve the success of each learner. To learn more, visit ASCD at http://www.ascd.org

For bulk orders: email us at trade.sales@cancer.org

National Health Education Standards
Review and Revision Panel

Steve Dorman, MPH, PhD, Chairman
University of Florida
College of Health and Human Performance

Jess Bogli, MS
Oregon Department of Education

Kim Robert Clark, MPH, DrPH, CHES
California State University–San Bernardino
Department of Health Science and Human
Ecology

Mary Connolly, BS, Med, CAGS
Cambridge College, Curry College
Massachusetts Department of Education

Marilyn Jensen, MA
University of South Dakota

Ellen Larson, MS, CHES
Northern Arizona University
Health Sciences Department

Mary Marks, PhD
California Department of Education
School Health Connections/Healthy Start

Antionette Meeks, EdD
Florida Department of Education
Coordinated School Health Program

Linda Morse, RN, MA
New Jersey Department of Education
Society of State Directors of Health Physical
Education and Recreation

Fred Peterson, PhD
The University of Texas at Austin
Department of Kinesiology & Health Education
American Public Health Association
School Health Education and Services Section

Eric Pliner
New York City Department of Education

Becky J. Smith, PhD, CHES
American Association for Health Education

Barbara Sullivan, BS, MS
Baltimore County Public Schools

Marlene K. Tappe, PhD, CHES
Minnesota State University, Mankato
Department of Health Science

Susan Telljohann, HSD, CHES
University of Toledo
Department of Public Health and Rehabilitative Services
American School Health Association

Valerie A. Ubbes, PhD, CHES
Miami University
Physical Education Health & Sport Studies

Mary Waters
American Cancer Society

Katherine Wilbur, MEd
Maine Department of Education
Coordinated School Health Programs
American Association for Health Education

Table of Contents

4 Assessment

Measuring Excellence

83

5 Background on Standards Development

A Background for Excellence

111

Glossary

117

A Vision of Excellence

Imagine a nation where children and adolescents are healthy, fit, and ready to learn; where youth are prepared with essential skills they need to live life to its fullest; where adult health and wellness are the natural outgrowth of skills, understanding, and behavior built from childhood; where health challenges, differences in ability, and socioeconomic disparities do not prevent our most precious human resources from reaching their potential.

Imagine a nation where children and adolescents are wise about the influences of technology and the media on their lives; where they are prepared to be prudent consumers of goods and services that enhance their health and well-being; where they are skilled in employing thoughtful decision-making and goal-setting strategies to achieve their greatest ambitions; where they passionately and compassionately advocate for the best for themselves, their families, and their communities.

We live in a time in which challenges to this vision come from forces surrounding our youth, our families, and our communities. There is unprecedented competition for our time, our attention, and our resources. Yet we also live in a time when the best thinking exists to move us in the right direction, a time when health education has dedicated itself to achieving this vision, a time when the vision will continue to move from existing as mere imagination to becoming an attainable goal for this generation of young people and for generations to come. Imagine. . . .

National Health Education Standards

1

Introduction

Prelude to Excellence

No knowledge is more crucial than knowledge about health.
Without it, no other life goal can be successfully achieved.

—Ernest Boyer, President,
The Carnegie Foundation for the
Advancement of Teaching
(1979–1995)

Developing Standards for Educational Excellence

I n the early 1990s, education leaders across the country agreed that schools needed new strategies, tools, and resources to support the highest levels of achievement by students in the United States. Following the lead of the National Education Goals (established in 1989 under President George H. W. Bush and a coalition of governors) and the "Goals 2000: Educate America" Act[1] (established under President William J. Clinton), the U.S. Department of Education funded the creation of model standards in the arts, civics and government, economics, English, foreign languages, geography, history, and science.

In response, a coalition of health education organizations and professionals from across the country was convened in July 1993 to write the National Health Education Standards (NHES). First published in 1995, the NHES were designed to support schools in meeting the essential goal of helping students acquire the knowledge and skills to promote personal, family, and community health.

A decade later, most states and many districts around the country had either adopted or adapted the NHES. Recognizing the critical role of schools in combating our nation's health problems while simultaneously acknowledging research-based advances related to effective practice in the field, a new panel of organizations and professionals was convened in 2004 to review and revise the NHES for use in American schools.

The revised NHES provide a framework for aligning curriculum, instruction, and assessment practices for the following groups, all of which play crucial roles in health instruction:

- State and local education agencies
- Education professionals
- Parents and families
- Community agencies, businesses, organizations, and institutions
- Health education curriculum developers and publishers
- Institutions of higher education
- Local and national organizations

Teachers, administrators, and policy makers can use the NHES as a framework for designing or selecting curricula, for allocating instructional resources, and for providing a basis for the assessment of student achievement and progress. The NHES also provide students, families, and communities with concrete expectations for health education. Although the standards identify what knowledge and skills students should have and be able to achieve, they leave precisely how this is to be accomplished to teachers and other local specialists who formulate, deliver, and evaluate curricula.

The revision of the NHES makes a number of important contributions to the potential for delivery of improved health education programs across the country, including increased focus on education and behavior theory, inclusion of pre-K grades, emphasis on assessment, and an expanded call for collaboration and partnerships.

Implementation of the revised NHES with a commitment to providing qualified teachers, adequate instructional time, and increased linkages to other school curricular areas significantly increases the likelihood that schools will provide high-quality health instruction to all young people.

Health Education as a Component of Coordinated School Health Programs

Health education is not the only school-based approach used to support students in attaining positive health outcomes. Health education is an essential component of a Coordinated School Health Program (CSHP) (**Fig. 1.1**), a planned, sequential, and integrated set of courses, services, policies, and interventions designed to meet the health and safety needs of students in kindergarten through grade 12.[2] One widely recognized model for CSHP consists of eight interactive components, each of which plays a vital role in supporting the health of students, school staff, and the community. In addition to health education, these components include physical education; health services; counseling, psychological, and social services; nutrition services; a healthy school environment; parent, family, and community involvement; and health promotion for school staff. The effectiveness of school health education is enhanced when it is implemented as part of a larger school health program and when health education outcomes are reinforced by the other components.

The NHES can be used to support the effective implementation of health education as one of the eight components of a CSHP. They are carefully designed to support schools, educators, families, and other stakeholders in helping students meet the primary goal of health education: for students to adopt and maintain healthy behaviors.

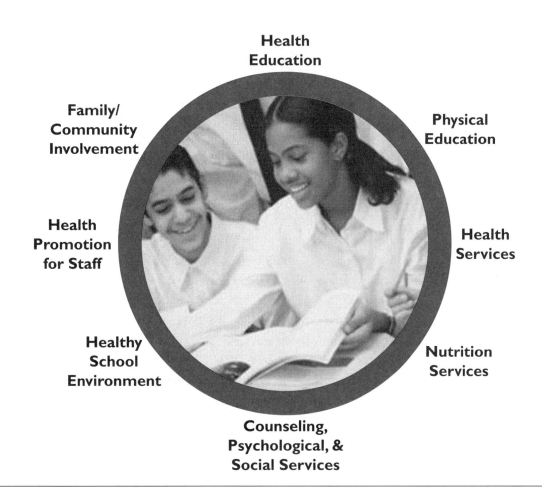

Figure 1.1 Coordinated School Health Programs, Centers for Disease Control and Prevention.[2]

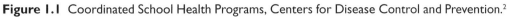

Adopting and Maintaining Healthy Behaviors: The Goal of Health Education

To help students adopt and maintain healthy behaviors, health education should contribute directly to a student's ability to successfully practice behaviors that protect and promote health and avoid or reduce health risks.

The educator's role in contributing to this goal includes the following:

- Teaching functional health information (essential concepts)
- Helping students determine personal values that support healthy behaviors
- Helping students develop group norms that value a healthy lifestyle
- Helping students develop the essential skills necessary to adopt, practice, and maintain health-enhancing behaviors

The NHES describe the knowledge and skills that are essential to the achievement of these factors. "Knowledge" includes the most important and enduring health education ideas and concepts. Essential "skills" encompass analysis and communication that lead to the practice and adoption of health-enhancing behaviors.

If the goal of health education is for students to adopt and maintain healthy behaviors, it is important that health educators have information about the behavioral outcomes on which to focus. While the NHES do not focus on specific behaviors, they provide a framework within which educators and curriculum specialists can focus on healthy behavior outcomes that are particular to the needs of their students.

In the development of the 1995 NHES, health literacy was accepted as the primary outcome of a comprehensive K–12 health education program. The Joint Committee on Health Education Terminology (1990) defined "health literacy" as "the capacity of an individual to obtain, interpret, and understand basic health information and services, and the competence to use such information and services in ways which are health enhancing."[3] A strong relationship continues to exist between goals of health literacy and school health education. The development of health literacy is presently considered to be essential for students to adopt and maintain healthy behaviors. A 2004 report by the Institute of Medicine on Health Literacy states that "the most effective means to improve health literacy is to ensure that education about health is part of the curriculum at all levels of education."[4]

The Scope of the National Health Education Standards: Parameters and Underlying Assumptions

In light of the role of health education as but one part of a student's learning during the school day, the development and revision of standards require maintenance of a clear, precise scope and focus. Before revising the NHES and accompanying performance indicators, the NHES Review and Revision Panel established parameters for its development and implementation. Specifically, the Panel determined that the revised NHES and performance indicators should accomplish the following:

- Provide a framework for curriculum development, instruction, and student assessment
- Reflect the research-based characteristics of effective health education
- Be informed by relevant health behavior theories and models

- Focus on personal health within the context of families, schools, and communities
- Focus on emotional, intellectual, physical, and social dimensions of health
- Focus on functional health knowledge and essential personal and social skills that contribute directly to healthy behaviors
- Focus on health promotion as well as avoidance and reduction of health risks
- Consider the developmental appropriateness of material for students in specific grade spans
- Include a progression of higher-order thinking skills
- Allow for the integration of health content as appropriate

Similarly, to establish consistency throughout the NHES document, the NHES Review and Revision Panel operated under the following set of assumptions, drawn from current theory and research in the field:

1. Academic achievement and the health status of students are interrelated.
2. All students, regardless of physical or intellectual ability, deserve the opportunity to achieve personal wellness.
3. Through the achievement of the NHES, students will adopt, practice, and maintain health-enhancing behaviors.
4. Instruction by qualified health education teachers is essential for student achievement of the NHES.
5. Sufficient instructional time is needed to influence the health behaviors of students through health instruction.
6. Health education emphasizes the teaching of functional health information and essential skills necessary to adopt, practice, and maintain health-enhancing behaviors.
7. Students need opportunities to engage in cooperative and active learning strategies, including practice and reinforcement of skills.
8. Health education encourages the use of technology to access multiple valid sources of health information.
9. Local curriculum planners should develop curricula based upon local health needs.
10. Students need multiple opportunities and a variety of assessment strategies to determine their achievement of the health standards and performance indicators.
11. Improvements in public health can contribute to a reduction in health care costs.
12. Effective health education can contribute to the establishment of a healthy and productive citizenry.

Following page: **Table 1.1** The National Health Education Standards

The National Health Education Standards

Standard 1:   Students will comprehend concepts related to health promotion and disease prevention to enhance health.

Standard 2:   Students will analyze the influence of family, peers, culture, media, technology, and other factors on health behaviors.

Standard 3:   Students will demonstrate the ability to access valid information and products and services to enhance health.

Standard 4:   Students will demonstrate the ability to use interpersonal communication skills to enhance health and avoid or reduce health risks.

Standard 5:   Students will demonstrate the ability to use decision-making skills to enhance health.

Standard 6:   Students will demonstrate the ability to use goal-setting skills to enhance health.

Standard 7:   Students will demonstrate the ability to practice health-enhancing behaviors and avoid or reduce health risks.

Standard 8:   Students will demonstrate the ability to advocate for personal, family, and community health.

A Closer Look at the Standards Document

The NHES document displays each standard (and its supporting information) as follows:

1. The standard
2. A rationale statement
3. Performance indicators (organized by grade span)

The Standards

Knowledge of core health concepts and underlying principles of health promotion and disease prevention are included in Standard 1. Standards 2 to 8 identify key processes and skills that are applicable to healthy living. These include identifying the impact of family, peers, culture, media, and technology on health behaviors; knowing how to access valid health information; using interpersonal communication, decision-making, goal-setting, and advocacy skills; and enacting personal health-enhancing practices (**Table 1.1**).

Rationale Statements

A rationale statement is provided for each standard. The rationale illustrates the importance of each standard and is intended to provide additional clarity, direction, and understanding.

Performance Indicators

Performance indicators are provided for each of the NHES, delineated by the following grade spans: pre-K to grade 2, grades 3 to 5, grades 6 to 8, and grades 9 to 12. Each performance indicator is introduced by this stem: "As a result of health instruction in [*grade range*], students will be able to . . ." The performance indicators are meant to be achieved by the end of the grade span in which they are identified.

Because learning best occurs when students perform at all levels of the cognitive domain, the performance indicators encompass application, analysis, synthesis, and evaluation, as well as knowledge and comprehension. Even primary grade students can learn at the higher levels of the cognitive domain if the concepts and learning activities are developmentally appropriate.

Performance indicators are also intended to serve as a blueprint for organizing student assessment. Student achievement of all performance indicators specified for each standard supports the successful attainment of that standard, ultimately increasing the likelihood that students will adopt and maintain healthy behaviors.

Building Curriculum: Integrating Health Content into the Standards and Performance Indicators

Historically, health education curricula were often organized around health content or topic areas. More recently, many health education curricula reflect the six priority adolescent risk behaviors identified by the U.S. Centers for Disease Control and Prevention. The object of the NHES is to provide a framework from which curricula can be developed, allowing for the inclusion of health content and concepts that are appropriate for local needs. This approach allows the NHES to remain relevant over time, and it enables state and local education agencies to determine the curriculum content that best addresses the state and local health needs of students.

Table 1.2 shows the relationship between the NHES and health content areas and risk behaviors. The standards are designed to encompass a wide range of content areas as well as promote healthy behaviors and decrease risky behaviors.

Many state education agencies will interpret the standards and provide further direction to local education agencies to assist them with development of specific curricula that meet national and state standards. In recognition of this process, the NHES do not address specific health education content areas; instead, they provide a framework from which curricula can be developed, allowing for the inclusion of health content appropriate to local needs. The selection of specific health content is left to state and local education agencies.

Table 1.3 shows how specific health content can be matched to selected performance indicators across the grade spans.

Common Health Education Content Areas	National Health Education Standards	Centers for Disease Control & Prevention Adolescent Risk Behaviors
• Community Health • Consumer Health • Environmental Health • Family Life • Mental/Emotional Health • Injury Prevention/Safety • Nutrition • Personal Health • Prevention/Control of Disease • Substance Use/Abuse	**Standard 1:** Students will comprehend concepts related to health promotion and disease prevention to enhance health. **Standard 2:** Students will analyze the influence of family, peers, culture, media, technology, and other factors on health behaviors. **Standard 3:** Students will demonstrate the ability to access valid information and products and services to enhance health. **Standard 4:** Students will demonstrate the ability to use interpersonal communication skills to enhance health and avoid or reduce health risks. **Standard 5:** Students will demonstrate the ability to use decision-making skills to enhance health. **Standard 6:** Students will demonstrate the ability to use goal-setting skills to enhance health. **Standard 7:** Students will demonstrate the ability to practice health-enhancing behaviors and avoid or reduce health risks. **Standard 8:** Students will demonstrate the ability to advocate for personal, family, and community health.	• Alcohol and Other Drug Use • Injury and Violence (Including Suicide) • Tobacco Use • Poor Nutrition • Inadequate Physical Activity • Risky Sexual Behavior

Table 1.2 Relationship of common health education content areas and Centers for Disease Control and Prevention adolescent risk behaviors to the National Health Education Standards.

Health Education Standard 1:

Students will comprehend concepts related to health promotion and disease prevention to enhance health.

Performance indicator (Pre-K–grade 2):
Identify that healthy behaviors affect personal health.

Examples:
- Identify that eating breakfast, lunch, and dinner helps keep the body healthy.
- Identify that regular physical activity helps keep the body healthy.

Performance indicator (grades 3–5):
Describe the relationship between healthy behaviors and personal health.

Examples:
- Describe the relationship between eating healthy foods and a healthy body.
- Describe the relationship between regular physical activity and a healthy heart.

Performance indicator (grades 6–8):
Analyze the relationship between healthy behavior and personal health.

Examples:
- Analyze the relationship between decreased intake of refined sugars and weight management.
- Analyze the relationship between cardiovascular exercise and stress management.

Performance indicator (grades 9–12):
Predict how healthy behaviors can affect health status.

Examples:
- Predict how adopting dietary practices recommended by the U.S. Department of Agriculture can affect health status.
- Predict how vigorous activity, as recommended by the Centers for Disease Control and Prevention, can affect health status.

Table 1.3 Example of Health Education Performance Indicators.

Characteristics of Effective Health Education Curricula

One of the key parameters of the NHES revision requires that the standards and performance indicators be based in research that identifies those characteristics of curricula that most positively influence students' health practices and behaviors. The Centers for Disease Control and Prevention, Division of Adolescent and School Health (CDC-DASH), has examined a synthesis of professional literature to determine the common characteristics of effective health education curricula. Reviews by CDC-DASH of effective programs and curricula, along with input from experts in the field of health education, have identified the following characteristics of effective health education curricula (many of which are reflected in the revised standards and performance indicators).[5-15]

An effective health education curriculum achieves the following:

- **Focuses on specific behavioral outcomes**
  Curricula have a clear set of behavioral outcomes. Instructional strategies and learning experiences focus exclusively on these outcomes.

- **Is research-based and theory-driven**
  Instructional strategies and learning experiences build on theoretical approaches, such as social cognitive theory and social inoculation theory, that have effectively influenced health-related behaviors among youth. The most promising curricula go beyond the cognitive level and address the social influences, attitudes, values, norms, and skills that influence specific health-related behaviors.

- **Addresses individual values and group norms that support health-enhancing behaviors**
  Instructional strategies and learning experiences help students accurately assess the level of risk-taking behavior among their peers (e.g., how many of their peers use illegal drugs), correct misperceptions of peer and social norms, and reinforce health-enhancing attitudes and beliefs.

- **Focuses on increasing the personal perception of risk and harmfulness of engaging in specific health risk behaviors, as well as reinforcing protective factors**
  Curricula provide opportunities for students to assess their actual vulnerability to health risk behaviors, health problems, and exposure to

unhealthy situations. Curricula also provide opportunities for students to affirm health-promoting beliefs, intentions, and behaviors.

- **Addresses social pressures and influences**
  Curricula provide opportunities for students to deal with relevant personal and social pressures that influence risky behaviors, such as the influence of the media, peer pressure, and social barriers.

- **Builds personal and social competence**
  Curricula build essential skills, including communication, refusal, assessing accuracy of information, decision making, planning, goal setting, and self-management, that enable students to build personal confidence and ability to deal with social pressures and avoid or reduce risk-taking behaviors. For each skill, students are guided through a series of developmental steps:

  1. Discussing the importance of the skill, its relevance, and its relationship to other learned skills
  2. Presenting steps for developing the skill
  3. Modeling the skill
  4. Practicing and rehearsing the skill by using real-life scenarios
  5. Providing feedback and reinforcement

- **Provides functional health knowledge that is basic, accurate, and directly contributes to health-promoting decisions and behaviors**
  Curricula provide accurate, reliable, and credible information for a usable purpose: so students can assess risk, correct misperceptions about social norms, identify ways to avoid or minimize risky situations, examine internal and external influences, make behaviorally relevant decisions, and build personal and social competence. A curriculum that relies exclusively or primarily on disseminating information for the sole purpose of improving knowledge is inadequate and incomplete.

- **Uses strategies designed to personalize information and engage students**
  Instructional strategies and learning experiences are student centered, interactive, and experiential. The strategies include group discussions, cooperative learning, problem solving, role playing, and peer-led activities. Learning experiences correspond with students' cognitive and emotional development and help them personalize information and maintain their interest and motivation while accommodating diverse capabilities and learning styles. Instructional strategies and learning experiences include

methods for the following:

1. Addressing key health-related concepts
2. Encouraging creative expression
3. Sharing personal thoughts, feelings, and opinions
4. Developing critical thinking skills

- **Provides age-appropriate and developmentally appropriate information, learning strategies, teaching methods, and materials**
  Curricula address students' needs, interests, concerns, developmental and emotional maturity, and current knowledge and skills. Learning should be relevant and applicable to students' daily lives.

- **Incorporates learning strategies, teaching methods, and materials that are culturally inclusive**
  Curricular materials are free of culturally biased information but also include information, activities, and examples that are inclusive of diverse cultures and lifestyles, such as gender, race, ethnicity, religion, age, physical/mental ability, and appearance. Strategies promote values, attitudes, and behaviors that support the cultural diversity of students; optimize relevance to students from multiple cultures in the school community; strengthen the skills that are necessary to engage in intercultural interactions; and build on the cultural resources of families and communities.

- **Provides adequate time for instruction and learning**
  Curricula use adequate time to promote understanding of key health concepts and to practice skills. Effecting change requires an intensive and sustained effort. Short-term or "one-shot" curricula (e.g., a few hours at one grade level) are generally insufficient to support the adoption and maintenance of healthy behaviors.

- **Provides opportunities to reinforce skills and positive health behaviors**
  Curricula build on previously learned concepts and skills and provide opportunities to reinforce health-promoting skills across health topic areas and grade levels, such as multiple practice applications of a skill and skill "booster" sessions at subsequent grade levels or in other academic subject areas. Curricula that address age-appropriate determinants of behavior across grade levels and reinforce and build on learning are more likely to achieve long-lasting results.

- **Provides opportunities to make connections with other influential persons**

   Curricula link students to other influential persons who affirm and reinforce health-promoting norms, beliefs, and behaviors. Instructional strategies build on protective factors that promote healthy behaviors and enable students to avoid or reduce health risk behaviors by engaging peers, parents, families, and other positive adult role models in student learning.

- **Includes teacher information and plans for professional development and training to enhance effectiveness of instruction and student learning**

   Curricula are implemented by teachers who have a personal interest in promoting positive health behaviors, believe in what they are teaching, are knowledgeable about the curriculum content, and are comfortable and skilled in implementing expected instructional strategies. Ongoing professional development and training are critical in helping teachers implement a new curriculum or implement strategies that require new skills in teaching or assessment.

Using the National Health Education Standards to Inform Development of Health Education Programs

The NHES provide a framework for curriculum development. They are not a curriculum, nor do they constitute objectives for a curriculum. The NHES and accompanying performance indicators describe what every student should know and be able to do upon completion of a grade span.

Included among the NHES are components of the essential knowledge and skills for the healthy development of children and adolescents. These standards are not, however, intended to be either restrictive or all-inclusive. State and local education agencies may develop ways to implement these standards. States and school districts may find that their local health needs require instruction that goes beyond the scope of the standards established herein. Whereas these standards have been carefully developed by expert panelists and have received wide approval by the field, state and district school organizations may choose to modify these standards to meet local or regional needs.

The NHES schematic (**Fig. 1.2**) provides a framework for understanding the relationship of the standards to other components of health education. Comprehensive school health education is one of the eight components of a CSHP model, as identified by CDC-DASH (see **Fig. 1.1**). The NHES and their accompanying performance indicators are designed to support the goals of

Characteristics of Effective Health Education

Effective Health Education:

- Focuses on specific behavioral outcomes

- Is research-based and theory-driven

- Addresses individual values & group norms that support health-enhancing behaviors

- Focuses on increasing personal perception of risk and harmfulness of engaging in specific health risk behaviors and reinforcing protective factors

- Addresses social pressures

- Builds personal and social competence

- Provides functional health knowledge that is basic, accurate, and directly contributes to health-promoting decisions & behaviors

- Uses strategies designed to personalize info & engage students

- Provides age- and developmentally appropriate information, learning strategies, teaching methods & materials

- Incorporates culturally inclusive learning strategies, teaching methods & materials

- Emphasizes adequate time for instruction

- Provides opportunities to reinforce skills & positive health behaviors

- Provides opportunities to make connections with other influential persons

- Includes teacher information & plans for professional development & training to enhance effectiveness of instruction and learning

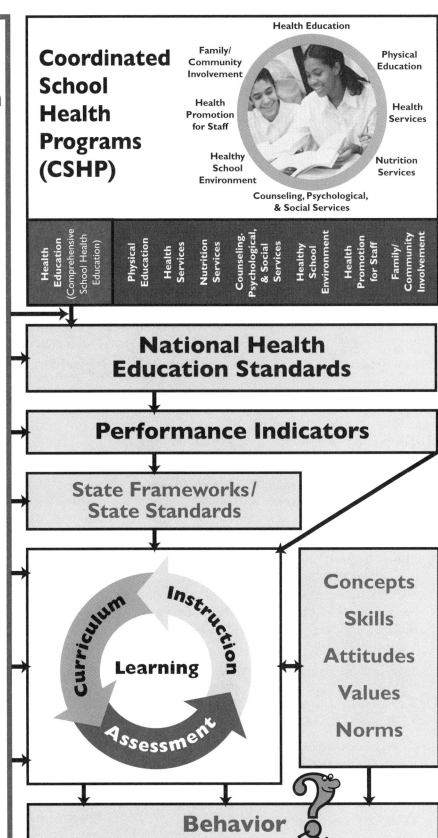

Coordinated School Health Programs (CSHP)

Health Education · Family/Community Involvement · Physical Education · Health Promotion for Staff · Health Services · Healthy School Environment · Nutrition Services · Counseling, Psychological, & Social Services

Health Education (Comprehensive School Health Education) · Physical Education · Health Services · Nutrition Services · Counseling, Psychological, & Social Services · Healthy School Environment · Health Promotion for Staff · Family/Community Involvement

National Health Education Standards

Performance Indicators

State Frameworks/State Standards

Curriculum · Instruction · Learning · Assessment

Concepts · Skills · Attitudes · Values · Norms

Behavior

Figure 1.2 Schematic for implementation of health education standards.

comprehensive school health education. From there, the NHES can and should be used to inform the development of state frameworks (ultimately helping to shape local curriculum) and/or to directly inform the design of local curriculum, instruction, and assessment—all of which should affect one another.

This local curriculum, instruction, and assessment should also be informed by the critical concepts, desired skills, intended attitudes, and community values and norms that schools would like students to understand and master. Health educators hope that the combination of these factors with carefully designed curriculum, instruction, and assessment will positively influence student health and/or risk behaviors.

Conversely, educators who seek to change existing negative student health and/or risk behaviors (as assessed by measures such as the Youth Risk Behavior Survey or community surveillance data) will allow those behaviors to inform priorities and content in the design of curriculum, instruction, and assessment tools. At all levels, the characteristics of effective health education (as documented by CDC-DASH) should be considered and, where appropriate, carefully incorporated into program design.

References

1. *Goals 2000: Educate America Act* (H.R. 1804). Accessed at http://www.ed.gov/legislation/GOALS2000/TheAct/index.html.

2. Centers for Disease Control and Prevention, National Center for Chronic Disease Prevention and Health Promotion. *Healthy Youth! Coordinated School Health Program*. Centers for Disease Control and Prevention, National Center for Chronic Disease Prevention and Health Promotion. Accessed at http://www.cdc.gov/healthyyouth/CSHP/.

3. American Association for Health Education. 2001. *Report of the 2000 Joint Committee on Health Education and Promotion Terminology*. Reston, VA: American Association for Health Education.

4. National Academy of Sciences. 2004. *Health Literacy: A Prescription to End Confusion*. 2004. Washington, D.C.: Institute of Medicine, National Academy of Sciences.

5. Botvin, G. J., E. M. Botvin, and H. Ruchlin. 1998. School-based approaches to drug abuse prevention: evidence for effectiveness and suggestions for determining cost-effectiveness. In *Cost-Benefit/ Cost-Effectiveness Research of Drug Abuse Prevention: Implications for Programming and Policy,* ed. W. J. Bukoski. Washington, D.C.: U.S. Department of Health and Human Services, pp. 59–82. Available at http://www.drugabuse.gov/pdf/monographs/monograph176/059-082_Botvin.pdf.

6. Contento, I., G. I. Balch, and Y. L. Bronner. 1995. Nutrition education for school-aged children. *Journal of Nutrition Education* 27:298–311.

7. Eisen, M., C. Pallitto, C. Bradner, and N. Bolshun. 2000. *Teen Risk-Taking: Promising Prevention Programs and Approaches*. Washington, D.C.: Urban Institute. Available at http://www.urban.org/MarvinEisen.

8. Gottfredson, D. C. 1998. School-based crime prevention. In *Preventing Crime: What Works, What Doesn't, What's Promising,* ed. L.W. Sherman, D. Gottfredson, D. MacKenzie, J. Eck, P. Reuter, and S. Bushway, National Institute of Justice. Available at http://www.ncjrs.org/pdffiles/171676.pdf.

9. Kirby, D. 2001. *Emerging Answers: Research Findings on Programs to Reduce Teen Pregnancy*. Washington, D.C.: National Campaign to Prevent Teen Pregnancy.

10. Lohrmann, D. K., and S. F. Wooley. 1998. Comprehensive school health education. In *Health Is Academic: A Guide to Coordinated School Health Programs,* ed. E. Marx and S. Wooley. New York: Teachers College Press, pp. 43–45.

11. Lytle, L., and C. Achterberg. 1995. Changing the diet of America's children: what works and why? *Journal of Nutrition Education* 27:250–60.

12. Stone, E. J., T. L. McKenzie, G. J. Welk, and M. L. Booth. 1998. Effects of physical activity interventions in youth. Review and synthesis. *American Journal of Preventive Medicine* 15:298–315.

13. Weed, S. E., and I. Ericksen. 2005. *A Model for Influencing Adolescent Sexual Behavior.* Salt Lake City, UT: Institute for Research and Evaluation. (Unpublished data.)

14. Symons, C. W., B. Cinelli, T. C. James, and P. Groff. 1997. Bridging student health risks and academic achievement through comprehensive school health programs. *Journal of School Health* 67:220–228.

15. Goldrick, L. 2000. *Improving Academic Performance by Meeting Student Health Needs.* Issue Brief, National Governors' Association Center for Best Practices, October 13, 2000.

2

The Standards

The Foundation for Excellence

The establishment of standards for the context of elementary and secondary education, student performance, and programs and services that enable students to achieve the content standards is at the heart of improving education in the United States. In addition to establishing these standards, it is essential to have benchmarks and indicators to monitor progress on student achievement and to judge the effectiveness and efficiency of schools. These benchmarks and indicators are important for informing the public and education decision-makers about key decisions affecting policy and practice and for accountability in the use of resources.

—The Coordinating Committee, State Education Improvement Partnership, CCSSO

National Health Education Standards— At a Glance

This chapter introduces the National Health Education Standards. The eight standards are presented, along with a rationale for each, and are followed by multiple performance indicators by grade span. The eight standards broadly and collectively articulate what students should know and be able to do to adopt or maintain health-enhancing behaviors.

The eight rationale statements support the importance of and provide additional clarity, direction, and understanding of each standard.

The performance indicators articulate specifically what students should *know* or *be able to do* in support of each standard by the conclusion of each of the following four grade spans:

- Pre-K through Grade 2
- Grade 3 through Grade 5
- Grade 6 through Grade 8
- Grade 9 through Grade 12

The standards, rationales, and performance indicators are first presented in order (standards 1 to 8). For ease of identification, the performance indicators are numbered sequentially.

Next, the standards and performance indicators are presented by each of the four grade spans.

Health Education Standard I

Students will comprehend concepts related to health promotion and disease prevention to enhance health.

RATIONALE

The acquisition of basic health concepts and functional health knowledge provides a foundation for promoting health-enhancing behaviors among youth. This standard includes essential concepts that are based on established health behavior theories and models. Concepts that focus on both health promotion and risk reduction are included in the performance indicators.

Health Education Standard 1 Performance Indicators

Pre-K–Grade 2

1.2.1   Identify that healthy behaviors affect personal health.
1.2.2   Recognize that there are multiple dimensions of health.
1.2.3   Describe ways to prevent communicable diseases.
1.2.4   List ways to prevent common childhood injuries.
1.2.5   Describe why it is important to seek health care.

Grades 3–5

1.5.1   Describe the relationship between healthy behaviors and personal health.
1.5.2   Identify examples of emotional, intellectual, physical, and social health.
1.5.3   Describe ways in which safe and healthy school and community environments can promote personal health.
1.5.4   Describe ways to prevent common childhood injuries and health problems.
1.5.5   Describe when it is important to seek health care.

(continued)

Health Education Standard 1 Performance Indicators *(continued)*

Grades 6–8

1.8.1	Analyze the relationship between healthy behaviors and personal health.
1.8.2	Describe the interrelationships of emotional, intellectual, physical, and social health in adolescence.
1.8.3	Analyze how the environment affects personal health.
1.8.4	Describe how family history can affect personal health.
1.8.5	Describe ways to reduce or prevent injuries and other adolescent health problems.
1.8.6	Explain how appropriate health care can promote personal health.
1.8.7	Describe the benefits of and barriers to practicing healthy behaviors.
1.8.8	Examine the likelihood of injury or illness if engaging in unhealthy behaviors.
1.8.9	Examine the potential seriousness of injury or illness if engaging in unhealthy behaviors.

Grades 9–12

1.12.1	Predict how healthy behaviors can affect health status.
1.12.2	Describe the interrelationships of emotional, intellectual, physical, and social health.
1.12.3	Analyze how environment and personal health are interrelated.
1.12.4	Analyze how genetics and family history can affect personal health.
1.12.5	Propose ways to reduce or prevent injuries and health problems.
1.12.6	Analyze the relationship between access to health care and health status.
1.12.7	Compare and contrast the benefits of and barriers to practicing a variety of healthy behaviors.
1.12.8	Analyze personal susceptibility to injury, illness, or death if engaging in unhealthy behaviors.
1.12.9	Analyze the potential severity of injury or illness if engaging in unhealthy behaviors.

Health Education Standard 2

Students will analyze the influence of family, peers, culture, media, technology, and other factors on health behaviors.

RATIONALE

Health is affected by a variety of positive and negative influences within society. This standard focuses on identifying and understanding the diverse internal and external factors that influence health practices and behaviors among youth, including personal values, beliefs, and perceived norms.

Health Education Standard 2 Performance Indicators

Pre-K–Grade 2

2.2.1	Identify how the family influences personal health practices and behaviors.
2.2.2	Identify what the school can do to support personal health practices and behaviors.
2.2.3	Describe how the media can influence health behaviors.

Grades 3–5

2.5.1	Describe how the family influences personal health practices and behaviors.
2.5.2	Identify the influence of culture on health practices and behaviors.
2.5.3	Identify how peers can influence healthy and unhealthy behaviors.
2.5.4	Describe how the school and community can support personal health practices and behaviors.
2.5.5	Explain how media influences thoughts, feelings, and health behaviors.
2.5.6	Describe ways that technology can influence personal health.

Grades 6–8

2.8.1	Examine how the family influences the health of adolescents.
2.8.2	Describe the influence of culture on health beliefs, practices, and behaviors.
2.8.3	Describe how peers influence healthy and unhealthy behaviors.

(continued)

Health Education Standard 2 Performance Indicators *(continued)*

2.8.4   Analyze how the school and community can affect personal health practices and behaviors.

2.8.5   Analyze how messages from media influence health behaviors.

2.8.6   Analyze the influence of technology on personal and family health.

2.8.7   Explain how the perceptions of norms influence healthy and unhealthy behaviors.

2.8.8   Explain the influence of personal values and beliefs on individual health practices and behaviors.

2.8.9   Describe how some health risk behaviors can influence the likelihood of engaging in unhealthy behaviors.

2.8.10   Explain how school and public health policies can influence health promotion and disease prevention.

Grades 9–12

2.12.1   Analyze how the family influences the health of individuals.

2.12.2   Analyze how the culture supports and challenges health beliefs, practices, and behaviors.

2.12.3   Analyze how peers influence healthy and unhealthy behaviors.

2.12.4   Evaluate how the school and community can affect personal health practice and behaviors.

2.12.5   Evaluate the effect of media on personal and family health.

2.12.6   Evaluate the impact of technology on personal, family, and community health.

2.12.7   Analyze how the perceptions of norms influence healthy and unhealthy behaviors.

2.12.8   Analyze the influence of personal values and beliefs on individual health practices and behaviors.

2.12.9   Analyze how some health risk behaviors can influence the likelihood of engaging in unhealthy behaviors.

2.12.10   Analyze how public health policies and government regulations can influence health promotion and disease prevention.

Health Education Standard 3

Students will demonstrate the ability to access valid information and products and services to enhance health.

RATIONALE

Access to valid health information and health-promoting products and services is critical in the prevention, early detection, and treatment of health problems. This standard focuses on how to identify and access valid health resources and to reject unproven sources. Application of the skills of analysis, comparison, and evaluation of health resources empowers students to achieve health literacy.

Health Education Standard 3 Performance Indicators

Pre-K–Grade 2

3.2.1   Identify trusted adults and professionals who can help promote health.

3.2.2   Identify ways to locate school and community health helpers.

Grades 3–5

3.5.1   Identify characteristics of valid health information, products, and services.

3.5.2   Locate resources from home, school, and community that provide valid health information

Grades 6–8

3.8.1   Analyze the validity of health information, products, and services.

3.8.2   Access valid health information from home, school, and community.

3.8.3   Determine the accessibility of products that enhance health.

3.8.4   Describe situations that may require professional health services.

3.8.5   Locate valid and reliable health products and services.

(continued)

Health Education Standard 3 Performance Indicators *(continued)*

Grades 9–12

3.12.1   Evaluate the validity of health information, products, and services.

3.12.2   Use resources from home, school, and community that provide valid health information.

3.12.3   Determine the accessibility of products and services that enhance health.

3.12.4   Determine when professional health services may be required.

3.12.5   Access valid and reliable health products and services.

Health Education Standard 4

*Students will demonstrate the ability to
use interpersonal communication skills to
enhance health and avoid or reduce health risks.*

RATIONALE

Effective communication enhances personal, family, and community health.
This standard focuses on how responsible individuals use verbal and nonverbal
skills to develop and maintain healthy personal relationships. The ability to
organize and convey information and feelings is the basis for strengthening
interpersonal interactions and reducing or avoiding conflict.

Health Education Standard 4 Performance Indicators

Pre-K–Grade 2

4.2.1	Demonstrate healthy ways to express needs, wants, and feelings.
4.2.2	Demonstrate listening skills to enhance health.
4.2.3	Demonstrate ways to respond when in an unwanted, threatening, or dangerous situation.
4.2.4	Demonstrate ways to tell a trusted adult if threatened or harmed.

Grades 3–5

4.5.1	Demonstrate effective verbal and nonverbal communication skills to enhance health.
4.5.2	Demonstrate refusal skills that avoid or reduce health risks.
4.5.3	Demonstrate nonviolent strategies to manage or resolve conflict.
4.5.4	Demonstrate how to ask for assistance to enhance personal health.

Grades 6–8

4.8.1	Apply effective verbal and nonverbal communication skills to enhance health.
4.8.2	Demonstrate refusal and negotiation skills that avoid or reduce health risks.
4.8.3	Demonstrate effective conflict management or resolution strategies.
4.8.4	Demonstrate how to ask for assistance to enhance the health of self and others.

(continued)

Health Education Standard 4 Performance Indicators *(continued)*

Grades 9–12

4.12.1 Use skills for communicating effectively with family, peers, and others to enhance health.

4.12.2 Demonstrate refusal, negotiation, and collaboration skills to enhance health and avoid or reduce health risks.

4.12.3 Demonstrate strategies to prevent, manage, or resolve interpersonal conflicts without harming self or others.

4.12.4 Demonstrate how to ask for and offer assistance to enhance the health of self and others.

Health Education Standard 5

Students will demonstrate the ability to use decision-making skills to enhance health.

RATIONALE

Decision-making skills are needed to identify, implement, and sustain health-enhancing behaviors. This standard includes the essential steps that are needed to make healthy decisions as prescribed in the performance indicators. When applied to health issues, the decision-making process enables individuals to collaborate with others to improve their quality of life.

Health Education Standard 5 Performance Indicators

Pre-K–Grade 2

5.2.1   Identify situations when a health-related decision is needed.

5.2.2   Differentiate between situations when a health-related decision can be made individually or when assistance is needed.

Grades 3–5

5.5.1   Identify health-related situations that might require a thoughtful decision.

5.5.2   Analyze when assistance is needed in making a health-related decision.

5.5.3   List healthy options to health-related issues or problems.

5.5.4   Predict the potential outcomes of each option when making a health-related decision.

5.5.5   Choose a healthy option when making a decision.

5.5.6   Describe the outcomes of a health-related decision.

Grades 6–8

5.8.1   Identify circumstances that can help or hinder healthy decision making.

5.8.2   Determine when health-related situations require the application of a thoughtful decision-making process.

5.8.3   Distinguish when individual or collaborative decision making is appropriate.

(continued)

Health Education Standard 5 Performance Indicators (continued)

5.8.4	Distinguish between healthy and unhealthy alternatives to health-related issues or problems.
5.8.5	Predict the potential short-term impact of each alternative on self and others.
5.8.6	Choose healthy alternatives over unhealthy alternatives when making a decision.
5.8.7	Analyze the outcomes of a health-related decision.

Grades 9–12

5.12.1	Examine barriers that can hinder healthy decision making.
5.12.2	Determine the value of applying a thoughtful decision-making process in health-related situations.
5.12.3	Justify when individual or collaborative decision making is appropriate.
5.12.4	Generate alternatives to health-related issues or problems.
5.12.5	Predict the potential short-term and long-term impact of each alternative on self and others.
5.12.6	Defend the healthy choice when making decisions.
5.12.7	Evaluate the effectiveness of health-related decisions.

Health Education Standard 6

Students will demonstrate the ability to use goal-setting skills to enhance health.

RATIONALE

Goal-setting skills are essential to help students identify, adopt, and maintain healthy behaviors. This standard includes the critical steps that are needed to achieve both short-term and long-term health goals. These skills make it possible for individuals to have aspirations and plans for the future.

Health Education Standard 6 Performance Indicators

Pre-K–Grade 2

6.2.1   Identify a short-term personal health goal and take action toward achieving the goal.

6.2.2   Identify who can help when assistance is needed to achieve a personal health goal.

Grades 3–5

6.5.1   Set a personal health goal and track progress toward its achievement.

6.5.2   Identify resources to assist in achieving a personal health goal.

Grades 6–8

6.8.1   Assess personal health practices.

6.8.2   Develop a goal to adopt, maintain, or improve a personal health practice.

6.8.3   Apply strategies and skills needed to attain a personal health goal.

6.8.4   Describe how personal health goals can vary with changing abilities, priorities, and responsibilities.

Grades 9–12

6.12.1   Assess personal health practices and overall health status.

6.12.2   Develop a plan to attain a personal health goal that addresses strengths, needs, and risks.

6.12.3   Implement strategies and monitor progress in achieving a personal health goal.

6.12.4   Formulate an effective long-term personal health plan.

Health Education Standard 7

Students will demonstrate the ability to practice health-enhancing behaviors and avoid or reduce health risks.

RATIONALE

Research confirms that the practice of health-enhancing behaviors can contribute to a positive quality of life. In addition, many diseases and injuries can be prevented by reducing harmful and risk-taking behaviors. This standard promotes the acceptance of personal responsibility for health and encourages the practice of healthy behaviors.

Health Education Standard 7 Performance Indicators

Pre-K–Grade 2

7.2.1   Demonstrate healthy practices and behaviors to maintain or improve personal health.

7.2.2   Demonstrate behaviors that avoid or reduce health risks.

Grades 3–5

7.5.1   Identify responsible personal health behaviors.

7.5.2   Demonstrate a variety of healthy practices and behaviors to maintain or improve personal health.

7.5.3   Demonstrate a variety of behaviors that avoid or reduce health risks.

Grades 6–8

7.8.1   Explain the importance of assuming responsibility for personal health behaviors.

7.8.2   Demonstrate healthy practices and behaviors that will maintain or improve the health of self and others.

7.8.3   Demonstrate behaviors that avoid or reduce health risks to self and others.

Grades 9–12

7.12.1   Analyze the role of individual responsibility in enhancing health.

7.12.2   Demonstrate a variety of healthy practices and behaviors that will maintain or improve the health of self and others.

7.12.3   Demonstrate a variety of behaviors that avoid or reduce health risks to self and others.

Health Education Standard 8

Students will demonstrate the ability to advocate for personal, family, and community health.

RATIONALE

Advocacy skills help students promote healthy norms and healthy behaviors. This standard helps students develop important skills to target their health-enhancing messages and to encourage others to adopt healthy behaviors.

Health Education Standard 8 Performance Indicators

Pre-K–Grade 2

8.2.1   Make requests to promote personal health.

8.2.2   Encourage peers to make positive health choices.

Grades 3–5

8.5.1   Express opinions and give accurate information about health issues.

8.5.2   Encourage others to make positive health choices.

Grades 6–8

8.8.1   State a health-enhancing position on a topic and support it with accurate information.

8.8.2   Demonstrate how to influence and support others to make positive health choices.

8.8.3   Work cooperatively to advocate for healthy individuals, families, and schools.

8.8.4   Identify ways in which health messages and communication techniques can be altered for different audiences.

Grades 9–12

8.12.1   Use accurate peer and societal norms to formulate a health-enhancing message.

8.12.2   Demonstrate how to influence and support others to make positive health choices.

8.12.3   Work cooperatively as an advocate for improving personal, family, and community health.

8.12.4   Adapt health messages and communication techniques to a specific target audience.

National Health Education Standards by Grade Span

For all eight standards, the performance indicators are the specific concepts and skills that students *should know* and *be able to do* by the end of grade 2.

Health Education Standard 1

Students will comprehend concepts related to health promotion and disease prevention to enhance health.

As a result of health instruction in grades pre-kindergarten through 2, students will

1.2.1   Identify that healthy behaviors affect personal health.
1.2.2   Recognize that there are multiple dimensions of health.
1.2.3   Describe ways to prevent communicable diseases.
1.2.4   List ways to prevent common childhood injuries.
1.2.5   Describe why it is important to seek health care.

Health Education Standard 2

Students will analyze the influence of family, peers, culture, media, technology and other factors on health behaviors.

As a result of health instruction in grades pre-kindergarten to 2, students will

2.2.1   Identify how the family influences personal health practices and behaviors.
2.2.2   Identify what the school can do to support personal health practices and behaviors.
2.2.3   Describe how the media can influence health behaviors.

Health Education Standard 3

Students will demonstrate the ability to access valid information and products and services to enhance health.

As a result of health instruction in grades pre-kindergarten through 2, students will

3.2.1   Identify trusted adults and professionals who can help promote health.

3.2.2   Identify ways to locate school and community health helpers.

Health Education Standard 4

Students will demonstrate the ability to use interpersonal communication skills to enhance health and avoid or reduce health risks.

As a result of health instruction in grades pre-kindergarten through 2, students will

4.2.1   Demonstrate healthy ways to express needs, wants, and feelings.

4.2.2   Demonstrate listening skills to enhance health.

4.2.3   Demonstrate ways to respond when in an unwanted, threatening, or dangerous situation.

4.2.4   Demonstrate ways to tell a trusted adult if threatened or harmed.

Health Education Standard 5

Students will demonstrate the ability to use decision-making skills to enhance health.

As a result of health instruction in grades pre-kindergarten through 2, students will

5.2.1   Identify situations when a health-related decision is needed.

5.2.2   Differentiate between situations when a health-related decision can be made individually or when assistance is needed.

Health Education Standard 6

Students will demonstrate the ability to use goal-setting skills to enhance health.

As a result of health instruction in grades pre-kindergarten through 2, students will

6.2.1   Identify a short-term personal health goal and take action toward achieving the goal.

6.2.2   Identify who can help when assistance is needed to achieve a personal health goal.

Health Education Standard 7

Students will demonstrate the ability to practice health-enhancing behaviors and avoid or reduce health risks.

As a result of health instruction in grades pre-kindergarten through 2, students will

7.2.1   Demonstrate healthy practices and behaviors that maintain or improve personal health.

7.2.2   Demonstrate behaviors that avoid or reduce health risks.

Health Education Standard 8

Students will demonstrate the ability to advocate for personal, family, and community health.

As a result of health instruction in grades pre-kindergarten through 2, students will

8.2.1   Make requests to promote personal health.

8.2.2   Encourage peers to make positive health choices.

GRADES 3–5

For all eight standards, the performance indicators are the specific concepts and skills that students *should know* and *be able to do* by the end of grade 5.

Health Education Standard 1

Students will comprehend concepts related to health promotion and disease prevention to enhance health.

As a result of health instruction in grades 3 through 5, students will

1.5.1   Describe the relationship between healthy behaviors and personal health.

1.5.2   Identify examples of emotional, intellectual, physical, and social health.

1.5.3   Describe ways in which safe and healthy school and community environments can promote personal health.

1.5.4   Describe ways to prevent common childhood injuries and health problems.

1.5.5   Describe when it is important to seek health care.

Health Education Standard 2

Students will analyze the influence of family, peers, culture, media, technology and other factors on health behaviors.

As a result of health instruction in grades 3 through 5, students will

2.5.1   Describe how the family influences personal health practices and behaviors.

2.5.2   Identify the influence of culture on health practices and behaviors.

2.5.3   Identify how peers can influence healthy and unhealthy behaviors.

2.5.4   Describe how the school and community can support personal health practices and behaviors.

2.5.5   Explain how media influences thoughts, feelings, and healthy behaviors.

2.5.6   Describe ways that technology can influence personal health.

Health Education Standard 3

*Students will demonstrate the ability to
access valid information and
products and services to enhance health.*

As a result of health instruction in grades 3 through 5, students will

3.5.1   Identify characteristics of valid health information, products, and services.

3.5.2   Locate resources from home, school, and community that provide valid health information.

Health Education Standard 4

*Students will demonstrate the ability to
use interpersonal communication skills to
enhance health and avoid or reduce health risks.*

As a result of health instruction in grades 3 through 5, students will

4.5.1   Demonstrate effective verbal and nonverbal communication skills to enhance health.

4.5.2   Demonstrate refusal skills that avoid or reduce health risks.

4.5.3   Demonstrate nonviolent strategies to manage or resolve conflict.

4.5.4   Demonstrate how to ask for assistance to enhance personal health.

Health Education Standard 5

*Students will demonstrate the ability to
use decision-making skills to enhance health.*

As a result of health instruction in grades 3 through 5, students will

5.5.1   Identify health-related situations that might require a thoughtful decision.

5.5.2   Analyze when assistance is needed when making a health-related decision.

5.5.3   List healthy options to health-related issues or problems.

5.5.4   Predict the potential outcomes of each option when making a health-related decision.

5.5.5   Choose a healthy option when making a decision.

5.5.6   Describe the outcomes of a health-related decision.

Health Education Standard 6

Students will demonstrate the ability to use goal-setting skills to enhance health.

As a result of health instruction in grades 3 through 5, students will

6.5.1   Set a personal health goal and track progress toward its achievement.

6.5.2   Identify resources to assist in achieving a personal health goal.

Health Education Standard 7

Students will demonstrate the ability to practice health-enhancing behaviors and avoid or reduce health risks.

As a result of health instruction in grades 3 through 5, students will

7.5.1   Identify responsible personal health behaviors.

7.5.2   Demonstrate a variety of healthy practices and behaviors to maintain or improve personal health.

7.5.3   Demonstrate a variety of behaviors that avoid or reduce health risks.

Health Education Standard 8

Students will demonstrate the ability to advocate for personal, family, and community health.

As a result of health instruction in grades 3 through 5, students will

8.5.1   Express opinions and give accurate information about health issues.

8.5.2   Encourage others to make positive health choices.

GRADES 6–8

For all eight standards, the performance indicators are the specific concepts and skills that students *should know* and *be able to do* by the end of grade 8.

Health Education Standard 1

Students will comprehend concepts related to health promotion and disease prevention to enhance health.

As a result of health instruction in grades 6 through 8, students will

1.8.1   Analyze the relationship between healthy behaviors and personal health.

1.8.2   Describe the interrelationships of emotional, intellectual, physical, and social health in adolescence.

1.8.3   Analyze how the environment affects personal health.

1.8.4   Describe how family history can affect personal health.

1.8.5   Describe ways to reduce or prevent injuries and other adolescent health problems.

1.8.6   Explain how appropriate health care can promote personal health.

1.8.7   Describe the benefits of and barriers to practicing healthy behaviors.

1.8.8   Examine the likelihood of injury or illness if engaging in unhealthy behaviors.

1.8.9   Examine the potential seriousness of injury or illness if engaging in unhealthy behaviors.

Health Education Standard 2

Students will analyze the influence of family, peers, culture, media, technology and other factors on health behaviors.

As a result of health instruction in grades 6 through 8, students will

2.8.1   Examine how the family influences the health of adolescents.

2.8.2   Describe the influence of culture on health beliefs, practices, and behaviors.

2.8.3   Describe how peers influence healthy and unhealthy behaviors.

2.8.4   Analyze how the school and community can affect personal health practices and behaviors.

2.8.5   Analyze how messages from media influence health behaviors.

2.8.6   Analyze the influence of technology on personal and family health.

2.8.7   Explain how the perceptions of norms influence healthy and unhealthy behaviors.

2.8.8   Explain the influence of personal values and beliefs on individual health practices and behaviors.

2.8.9   Describe how some health risk behaviors can influence the likelihood of engaging in unhealthy behaviors.

2.8.10 Explain how school and public health policies can influence health promotion and disease prevention.

Health Education Standard 3

Students will demonstrate the ability to access valid information and products and services to enhance health.

As a result of health instruction in grades 6 through 8, students will

3.8.1   Analyze the validity of health information, products, and services.

3.8.2   Access valid health information from home, school, and community.

3.8.3   Determine the accessibility of products that enhance health.

3.8.4   Describe situations that may require professional health services.

3.8.5   Locate valid and reliable health products and services.

Health Education Standard 4

Students will demonstrate the ability to use interpersonal communication skills to enhance health and avoid or reduce health risks.

As a result of health instruction in grades 6 through 8, students will

4.8.1   Apply effective verbal and nonverbal communication skills to enhance health.

4.8.2   Demonstrate refusal and negotiation skills that avoid or reduce health risks.

4.8.3   Demonstrate effective conflict management or resolution strategies.

4.8.4   Demonstrate how to ask for assistance to enhance the health of self and others.

Health Education Standard 5

Students will demonstrate the ability to use decision-making skills to enhance health.

As a result of health instruction in grades 6 through 8, students will

5.8.1   Identify circumstances that can help or hinder healthy decision making.

5.8.2   Determine when health-related situations require the application of a thoughtful decision-making process.

5.8.3   Distinguish when individual or collaborative decision making is appropriate.

5.8.4   Distinguish between healthy and unhealthy alternatives to health-related issues or problems.

5.8.5   Predict the potential short-term impact of each alternative on self and others.

5.8.6   Choose healthy alternatives over unhealthy alternatives when making a decision.

5.8.7   Analyze the outcomes of a health-related decision.

Health Education Standard 6

Students will demonstrate the ability to use goal-setting skills to enhance health.

As a result of health instruction in grades 6 through 8, students will

6.8.1   Assess personal health practices.

6.8.2   Develop a goal to adopt, maintain, or improve a personal health practice.

6.8.3   Apply strategies and skills needed to attain a personal health goal.

6.8.4   Describe how personal health goals can vary with changing abilities, priorities, and responsibilities.

Health Education Standard 7

Students will demonstrate the ability to practice health-enhancing behaviors and avoid or reduce health risks.

As a result of health instruction in grades 6 through 8, students will

7.8.1 Explain the importance of assuming responsibility for personal health behaviors.

7.8.2 Demonstrate healthy practices and behaviors that will maintain or improve the health of self and others.

7.8.3 Demonstrate behaviors that avoid or reduce health risks to self and others.

Health Education Standard 8

Students will demonstrate the ability to advocate for personal, family and community health.

As a result of health instruction in grades 6 through 8, students will

8.8.1 State a health-enhancing position on a topic and support it with accurate information.

8.8.2 Demonstrate how to influence and support others to make positive health choices.

8.8.3 Work cooperatively to advocate for healthy individuals, families, and schools.

8.8.4 Identify ways that health messages and communication techniques can be altered for different audiences.

GRADES 9–12

For all eight standards, the performance indicators are the specific concepts and skills that students *should know* and *be able to do* by the end of grade 12.

Health Education Standard 1

Students will comprehend concepts related to health promotion and disease prevention to enhance health.

As a result of health instruction in grades 9 through 12, students will

1.12.1   Predict how healthy behaviors can affect health status.

1.12.2   Describe the interrelationships of emotional, intellectual, physical, and social health.

1.12.3   Analyze how environment and personal health are interrelated.

1.12.4   Analyze how genetics and family history can affect personal health problems.

1.12.5   Propose ways to reduce or prevent injuries and health problems.

1.12.6   Analyze the relationship between access to health care and health status.

1.12.7   Compare and contrast the benefits of and barriers to practicing a variety of health behaviors.

1.12.8   Analyze personal susceptibility to injury, illness, or death if engaging in unhealthy behaviors.

1.12.9   Analyze the potential severity of injury or illness if engaging in unhealthy behaviors.

Health Education Standard 2

Students will analyze the influence of family, peers, culture, media, technology and other factors on health behaviors.

As a result of health instruction in grades 9 through 12, students will

2.12.1   Analyze how the family influences the health of individuals.

2.12.2   Analyze how the culture supports and challenges health beliefs, practices, and behaviors.

2.12.3   Analyze how peers influence healthy and unhealthy behaviors.

2.12.4   Evaluate how the school and community can affect personal health practice and behaviors.

2.12.5   Evaluate the effect of media on personal and family health.

2.12.6   Evaluate the impact of technology on personal, family, and community health.

2.12.7   Analyze how the perceptions of norms influence healthy and unhealthy behaviors.

2.12.8   Analyze the influence of personal values and beliefs on individual health practices and behaviors.

2.12.9   Analyze how some health risk behaviors can influence the likelihood of engaging in unhealthy behaviors.

2.12.10 Analyze how public health policies and government regulations can influence health promotion and disease prevention.

Health Education Standard 3

Students will demonstrate the ability to access valid information and products and services to enhance health.

As a result of health instruction in grades 9 through 12, students will

3.12.1   Evaluate the validity of health information, products, and services.

3.12.2   Use resources from home, school, and community that provide valid health information.

3.12.3   Determine the accessibility of products and services that enhance health.

3.12.4   Determine when professional health services may be required.

3.12.5   Access valid and reliable health products and services.

Health Education Standard 4

Students will demonstrate the ability to use interpersonal communication skills to enhance health and avoid or reduce health risks.

As a result of health instruction in grades 9 through 12, students will

4.12.1   Use skills for communicating effectively with family, peers, and others to enhance health.

4.12.2   Demonstrate refusal, negotiation, and collaboration skills to enhance health and avoid or reduce health risks.

4.12.3   Demonstrate strategies to prevent, manage, or resolve interpersonal conflicts without harming self or others.

4.12.4   Demonstrate how to ask for and offer assistance to enhance the health of self and others.

Health Education Standard 5

Students will demonstrate the ability to use decision-making skills to enhance health.

As a result of health instruction in grades 9 through 12, students will

5.12.1   Examine barriers that can hinder healthy decision making.

5.12.2   Determine the value of applying a thoughtful decision-making process in health-related situations.

5.12.3   Justify when individual or collaborative decision making is appropriate.

5.12.4   Generate alternatives to health-related issues or problems.

5.12.5   Predict the potential short-term and long-term impact of each alternative on self and others.

5.12.6   Defend the healthy choice when making decisions.

5.12.7   Evaluate the effectiveness of health-related decisions.

Health Education Standard 6

Students will demonstrate the ability to use goal-setting skills to enhance health.

As a result of health instruction in grades 9 through 12, students will

6.12.1   Assess personal health practices and overall health status.

6.12.2   Develop a plan to attain a personal health goal that addresses strengths, needs, and risks.

6.12.3   Implement strategies and monitor progress in achieving a personal health goal.

6.12.4   Formulate an effective long-term personal health plan.

Health Education Standard 7

Students will demonstrate the ability to practice health-enhancing behaviors and avoid or reduce health risks.

As a result of health instruction in grades 9 through 12, students will

7.12.1   Analyze the role of individual responsibility for enhancing health.

7.12.2   Demonstrate a variety of healthy practices and behaviors that will maintain or improve the health of self and others.

7.12.3   Demonstrate a variety of behaviors that avoid or reduce health risks to self and others.

Health Education Standard 8

Students will demonstrate the ability to advocate for personal, family, and community health.

As a result of health instruction in grades 9 through 12, students will

8.12.1   Use accurate peer and societal norms to formulate a health-enhancing message.

8.12.2   Demonstrate how to influence and support others to make positive health choices.

8.12.3   Work cooperatively as an advocate for improving personal, family, and community health.

8.12.4   Adapt health messages and communication techniques to specific target audience.

3

Access and Equity Principles

Opportunities for Achieving Excellence

---

*We must agree to identify and employ initiatives that hold the greatest promise
for moving all students—including students of color, poor students, rural and urban students,
and second-language learners—to high levels of achievement.*

—GINA BURKHARDT, CEO, Learning Point Associates

Health Education
Access and Equity Principles

Access to an equitable, high-quality health education program is necessary for student attainment of the National Health Education Standards (NHES). The NHES provide states and local education agencies with direction for an effective instructional program, but it is the responsibility of educational institutions and their partners to provide all students with opportunities to learn the content and skills outlined in the standards. The following section provides the following:

- An explanation of the need for access and equity in health education
- An overview of the factors that impact student achievement
- A chart of the Access and Equity Principles that will address those factors
- Narratives of each of the Access and Equity Principles (Environment and Climate, Teaching, Curriculum, Assessment, Technology, and Learning)
- An explanation of the role of partners in supporting quality health education through access and equity for all students
- A charting of the action steps that each partner (local education agencies; state education agencies; institutions of higher education; national organizations and agencies; community agencies, organizations, institutions, and businesses; and families and caregivers) can take to address the Access and Equity Principles

It is the intent of the NHES that *all* students learn to make safe, appropriate, and healthful choices. "*All* students" necessitates access to instruction, which must not be denied for any reason. Health instruction should not be sacrificed to other educational variables, nor should it be provided in a way that reduces its value. Access should not be relegated only to those students who have room in their schedule or to students perceived to be at high risk for unhealthy behaviors. "*All* students" includes those who are college-bound or career-bound, students who are academically talented, students whose native language is not English, students with disabilities, and students from diverse socioeconomic backgrounds.

Even the best standards cannot ensure that all students will learn the essential concepts and skills embodied in them. Gaps in learning achievement occur in great part as a result of implementation. Four factors have been identified as key to the student achievement gap: access to a challenging curriculum, expectations of and from students, access to quality teaching, and equitable distribution of resources.[1]

These factors profoundly influence student capacity to learn and achieve the essential concepts and skills of the NHES. Therefore, it is important for students to receive an instructional program that is—

- grounded in a well-developed, cohesive, and current curriculum;
- provided by highly qualified (and appropriately licensed/certified) health teachers who use effective research-based classroom strategies to teach both knowledge and skills;
- guided by effective assessment of students, needs, knowledge, and skills; and
- supported with the time and resources necessary to accomplish learning and accommodate differences.

To accomplish this, six areas—(1) Environment and Climate, (2) Teaching, (3) Curriculum, (4) Assessment, (5) Technology, and (6) Learning—have been identified as health education Access and Equity Principles, which influence the effective implementation of the NHES. They describe the necessary actions to ensure that health education is of a quality that—

- all students will perceive it is valued as a component of the educational mission of the school and therefore is of value to learn, and
- all students will be provided with the instructional guidance, resources, support, and time necessary to acquire functional knowledge and to practice skills and processes to influence health behavior.

The Principles address equity in two contexts: (1) health education as a program to be provided for all students in a fair and impartial manner, and (2) health education for all students as an essential part of the school's mission. Excellence in any aspect of education requires equity. "Equity and excellence are mutually supportive values which should be applied to any decision made that affects life in public schools. The key questions for those who are making decisions that affect schools are these: Is it just? Is it fair? Is it reasonable? Is it theoretically and empirically defensible? Is it right?"[2] These questions need to be answered by decision makers and collaborative partners regarding the degree of equity and level of excellence that are expected of and therefore delivered within a school's health education program.

The Principles serve as a guide or tool for decision makers and collaborative partners to address the development, implementation, evaluation, and support of a rigorous and relevant health education program for all students. When supported, the Principles will ensure effective program implementation and support of instruction grounded in the NHES.

Schools are preparing students for a world of globalization, with demographic, technological, and health care issues that are not yet fully understood. What we envision for our children's future determines the educational tools we see fit to give them. It is advantageous for their future—and ours—to value their health and increase their capacity to adopt and maintain health practices and behaviors that will enable them to be proactive as well as resilient in an ever-changing world. The Principles, outlined in **Table 3.1**, provide the guidance that is needed to help accomplish this in an equitable fashion.

The Environment and Climate Principle

Schools are responsible for providing a healthful and safe school environment that optimizes opportunities for learning and growth. When the health of children and thus the desire that children be educated to build personal health capacity are valued, the climate and environment will be supportive of instruction grounded in the NHES.

The Environment and Climate Principle addresses the physical, social, emotional, and intellectual climate of the school community and the role that various partners play to support a safe, nurturing environment conducive to learning. According to Healthy People 2010,[3] schools have more influence on the lives of young people than any other social institution, except for the family, and provide a setting in which friendship networks develop, socialization occurs, and behavioral norms are developed and reinforced. To this end, schools should provide students the opportunity to acquire health-enhancing knowledge and skills to participate successfully in their own development. Supportive environmental conditions not only address health instruction but facilitate healthy choices to protect a student's well-being. For example, the serving of healthful foods as part of the school food services program reinforces what students learn in health class about healthful eating.

A learning environment conducive to health education would be equitable with other valued disciplines and would include—

- health education as a required program of study;
- inclusion of health education as a subject on student progress reports;
- scheduling and class sizes that demonstrate a commitment to the acquisition of functional health knowledge and skills;
- the assignment of licensed/certified teachers who have a deep understanding of health pedagogy and who would establish a classroom environment that would optimize student attainment of the NHES;
- a designated health education classroom, which would provide easy access to texts, technology, and student resources within the room; allow sensitive instructional materials to be maintained in a specific area; provide the opportunity for health materials, models, and student work to be

Table 3.1 Access and Equity Principles at a Glance

Principle	Description
Environment and Climate	All students will have access to facilities that are conducive to learning. An equitable learning environment in health education includes the physical classroom, resources, and tools for learning that would be equivalent to those in other subject areas. It also includes a school climate that values student health and safety as important tenets of education and regards instruction in these subjects as necessary to the development of the total child.
Teaching	All students will have access to competent delivery of health instruction. Teachers will have strong health education pedagogy skills, a passion for teaching about health, and compassion for students. Health educators will facilitate student-centered learning that engages students in real-world application of content. Teaching will be meaningful, equitable, rigorous, and relevant, providing all students with the opportunity to understand health concepts and apply them to the performance of health-enhancing skills.
Curriculum	All students will have access to a Pre-K–grade 12 health education instructional program guided by a curriculum grounded in the NHES. The curriculum will outline what students must know and be able to do. It will have well-defined scope and sequence that are developmentally appropriate and skill-based. It will be equitable and applicable, providing for meaningful instruction by addressing the diverse health issues and learning styles of students.
Assessment	All students will have access to assessment that accurately measures what they know and are able to do. Student achievement of standards will be assessed. Teachers will select and/or develop items and tasks that are equitable and fairly assess student performance. Assessments will be aligned with the curriculum and its implementation, employ multiple formats based on cognitive demand, and inform instruction.
Technology	All students will have access to technology to explore, analyze, and communicate about health issues, because competence in the use of technology as a consumer health tool is essential. Technology can and will influence what and how health education is taught, opening the door to real-world applications and enhancing student learning. The opportunity for technological experiences in health instruction and therefore the provision of technology resources will be consistent with opportunities provided in other subject areas.
Learning	All students will have access to programs that enable learning with behavioral intent. The goal of health education is the transference of understanding into healthy behaviors. Learning requires time and effort; therefore, adequate instructional time for skill development will be provided. Learning is best achieved with application that builds on prior knowledge; therefore, programs will be relevant, enhancing students' personal investment in their learning. Learning opportunities will be equitable but differentiated to meet the cognitive and behavioral needs of all students.

displayed and viewed; and allow teachers to reconfigure student desks to meet instructional and learning needs; and

- health education as a contributing component of coordinated school health efforts.

Health education not only optimally improves the health and safety of students; it also enhances the school learning environment. Student skill attainment manifested in healthy behaviors will contribute to the safe and orderly functioning of a school. Those behaviors may also enhance a student's capacity to address personal health and safety issues that may inhibit his or her ability to come to school ready to learn. No other standards provide the capacity to contribute so directly to the overall environment and mission of a school.

The Teaching Principle

Teaching is a dynamic human endeavor. Although it is very important that health education teachers know the content and pedagogy of their discipline, most student learning grows out of a relationship with teachers who know how to organize and plan lessons in a variety of ways. Teachers who plan only one way for their students to access health-related knowledge and skills can be effective. However, teachers who plan a variety of entry points[4] for a health lesson have more success in meeting the diverse and changing needs of their students. Health education teachers who value relationships with their students will understand ways to adapt core concepts and skills so that health lessons will be culturally and developmentally appropriate, gender sensitive, and academically sound.

Teaching requires an ongoing process of assessing the prior knowledge, individual talents, and abilities of pre-K–12 students; planning learning episodes to meet the individual and collective needs of diverse students; and then implementing and determining the effectiveness of the sequenced lessons. Quality or master teachers know how to use student work samples to evaluate their teaching, because effective teaching is based on the learning outcomes of students. If students are not learning, then the teaching planning process must include a revision and re-teaching phase so that students will be able to know health-related information, practice health-related skills, and demonstrate health-related behaviors on a consistent basis.

Learners move between school, home, and community contexts. Health teachers must know how to present concepts and skills so that the targeted health outcomes are reinforced and practiced during class and beyond. Teachers are responsible for the learning that occurs in their classrooms, but they can also be conduits for health-related messages, lessons, and programs that target healthful skill development for children and youth across the pre-K–12

Effective schools provide a safe and orderly learning environment.

—Robert J. Marzano, *What Works in Schools: Translating Research into Action*

Access and Equity Principles

curriculum. In this regard, health educators can be teacher-leaders who advocate for ongoing changes in school wellness policies and health instructional practices that result in improved learning experiences for children and youth.

Effective teachers help reduce barriers to learning by using brain-based instructional strategies[5] and by motivating students through relevant and engaging assignments. An expert teacher knows how to support the intellectual growth and development of students without taking over the thinking process for them. This requires that teachers know how to use concrete examples and exercises in abstract thinking, can recognize how students construct understanding from their prior knowledge and ongoing experiences, and are able to motivate learners through solo and cooperative/group experiences. Effective health education teachers also teach students through observation, analysis, and discussion, including the use of media and various technologies to capture student interest. Teaching health-related concepts and skills involves distinguishing between facts and fallacies and uncovering misconceptions of what students know and do. Health education teachers who focus on a variety of assessments will be able to support the ongoing growth and development of their students.

The Curriculum Principle

"Whether one advocates developing focused curriculum with 'backward design'—beginning with the final product or assessment and determining what is necessary for students to do to arrive there successfully—or one advocates specifying the essentials up front and moving ahead, clarity of design is the goal."[6] A focused curriculum is outlined with learning goals that are known by both teachers and students alike. The NHES are an example of learning goals that clarify the design of health education curricula.

When planning what students will know and be able to do, the curriculum designer or the teacher who plans the sequenced lessons for a specific grade level must be aware of the *scope* of health-related concepts and skills and the developmental *sequence* of lessons over time. Of the three types of curricula in health education—e.g., comprehensive, categorical, and integrated[7]—comprehensive curricula afford schools the advantage of a common language and skill set that is articulated between student grade levels and teacher lesson plans from school to school across a district. Regardless of which curriculum is selected or developed for implementation, the scope and sequence of lessons should be aligned to the NHES to outline what students should know and be able to do throughout their pre-K–12 schooling experience.

A health education curriculum "should be comprehensive, providing a wide range of information related to adolescent health and health-related behaviors. It should also help students develop their skills in risk assessment, decision-making, and communication."[8] The curriculum should provide a balanced representation of cultures and groups; and individuals and situations must be represented without bias and stereotypes.[9]

As summarized by the Centers for Disease Control and Prevention, Division of Adolescent and School Health, "health education curriculum includes those materials and experiences delivered in the classroom setting that provide students with opportunities to acquire the attitudes, knowledge and skills necessary for making health-promoting decisions, achieving health literacy, and adopting health-enhancing behaviors."[10] Students participating in a formal health education class have the opportunity to practice health-enhancing skills.[11]

In its simplest form, a standards-based curriculum is a plan for teaching. A health education curriculum outlines what content will be taught, e.g., concepts and skills, and the instructional strategies for teaching pre-K–12 students about personal health. Characteristics of effective health education curricula are discussed in Chapter 1.

Effective health education curricula must be reviewed, analyzed, and implemented on a local level with the intent to teach them as they were designed. When implemented with fidelity, the evidence-based curricula may hold up in different contexts as long as additional research data are collected to assess whether a curriculum made a difference with students in the new context. With any curriculum implementation, teachers learn to make local adaptations for their students who learn at a faster pace or are ready for greater depth or breadth, have difficulty learning, are just learning to speak English, have cultural or gender learning preferences, or who have given up on school.[6]

To be sensitive to the diverse needs and backgrounds of students, health education curricula must be accessible to all learners. School administrators must continue to support equitable time and funding for the development, alignment, purchase, and use of health education curricula, resources, and materials so that *all* students have the opportunity to learn.

The Assessment Principle

Assessment, a key component in the delivery of health instruction, contributes significantly to student comprehension and application of health-enhancing behaviors and skills. Whether and how students apply this learning in their everyday lives is the true summative assessment of their ability to enhance their health. It is therefore essential that students be provided with authentic assessment that is equitable and accomplished through multiple opportunities within the health education classroom. Ensuring that *all* students are appropriately assessed in the achievement of the NHES is paramount to student success.

Research has identified challenging goals and effective feedback as key elements of school effectiveness.[12] This requires that schools, teachers, parents/caregivers, and community leaders have high expectations for all students, conduct regular reviews of goals, and create a system of feedback regarding the achievement of those goals. Student achievement is at the core of goal expectations and must be effectively measured. Assessing student achievement provides teachers with the information and feedback necessary to adapt or revise instruction to meet student needs. Accurate assessment often requires that teachers make adaptations of time, resources, and formats to meet particular student needs. In addition, assessment provides students with feedback that is essential to determine their level of performance and course of action.

Health education requires that information be internalized to become personal. Providing all students with the opportunity to learn in health education must include occasions to assess their personal behaviors and competency to enhance their health. Therefore, equity in assessment in health education demands that assessments be fair, impartial, and realistic with regard to the issues, concerns, resources, and capabilities of the students served. It is essential that students have access to rigorous assessment and that they be provided with the instructional time to develop and process performance products that reflect deeper understanding and provide the opportunity for personal application.

All students, regardless of their ethnicity, background, learning abilities, and physical challenges, must acquire functional health knowledge and skills and be effectively assessed on their ability to apply this learning. Assessments should address goals and objectives that are aligned with NHES. Items that are selected or developed by a teacher must be clearly written at an appropriate reading level, culturally and developmentally appropriate, engaging, and authentic. It would be unrealistic, for example, for students to be given a decision-making role play with a sentence that begins, "Your parents are on a yachting trip . . ." when many students have no concept of a yacht. Assessment should provide for application of relevant skills, accommodate various learning styles, and clearly evaluate what students know and are able to do regarding their health and safety.[13]

Finally, assessment drives instruction. Without access to high-quality assessment and equity in implementation, teachers will not gain the necessary insights to move students to the next level in their acquisition of health-enhancing behaviors and skills.

The Technology Principle

Technology encompasses the tools and strategies for solving problems, using information, increasing productivity, and enhancing personal growth. It is an essential tool in the development of health literacy. To provide health instruction without the benefit of technology diminishes students' capacity for rigor and relevance and negatively affects learning outcomes. In the future, information technology will continue to evolve into new modes of communication and processing, biotechnology will continue to make advances in biological sciences and practical applications, and nanotechnology will continue to create new and more concise tools and processes.[14] As these fields evolve and merge, advancements in technology will give rise to ethical, medical, and consumer issues in health, which will require the attention and application of a public that is wise about health.

The goal of technology within the context of health education is to help students live, learn, and work successfully and responsibly in an increasingly complex, technology-driven society. Research on the transfer of learning strongly supports the position that instruction and educational activities should closely parallel the final desired behavior. The measure of the effectiveness of technologies and technology-enhanced educational programs is the extent to which they promote and support students' engaged learning and collaboration. The twenty-first-century citizen must be able to learn and respond in a rapidly changing environment, with skills to think critically and strategically to solve problems. The effective use of technology promotes—

- engaged, meaningful learning and collaboration involving challenging and real-life skills, and
- technology as a tool for learning, communication, and collaboration.

Access

There are two issues regarding access to technology in health education: (1) access to assistive technologies that will enable all students to participate in health education and (2) access to technology-based instruction and tools as an integral component of a student's experience within the health education curriculum. Access to technology to enhance and extend the delivery of health education must be equitable. Provision of fewer opportunities than in other subjects would promulgate and extend differences in educational quality and resources among content areas.

Equity

Technology is a tool that gives everyone an equal chance to learn. Given its significance in national and local policy, all students in all schools and within all content areas (including health education) should have equitable access to technology in ways that support engaged learning. As schools and districts continue to integrate technology into instruction, one of their overriding goals must be to adopt plans and policies that support this. Appropriate funding for technological resources and professional development for health teachers are key elements in the equitable application of technology to support meaningful learning for all students.

Within the health education classroom, teachers who engage students through authentic uses of technology provide students with opportunities to interact with a wealth of resources, materials, and data sets. When educational technology applications such as the Internet, distance learning, and digital media are used at the classroom level to help achieve challenging health education standards, more global alternatives are available for creating effective and productive learning environments.

To assess the extent of technological access and equity, schools and districts should ask the following questions: How does the distribution of educational technology (both amount and type) among classrooms or among schools affect equity of access and use? In what ways do equitable access and use depend upon the total amount of funding available to schools for purchases, installation, and operation of educational technology? In what ways do the ease and availability of technology, as well as professional development opportunities, affect the equitable access and use of education technology by students?

The Learning Principle

Learning requires time and effort. The goal of health education is the transference of knowledge and skills into health-enhancing behaviors. When schools do not devote enough time to implementing health education lessons and curricula in a planned and sequenced way, students are left with gaps in their health knowledge and skills. Mastery of skills requires wanting to learn because the skill is personally important, observing how and when the skill is used effectively, having the steps to the skill broken down and modeled, and practicing the skill toward eventual mastery.

Learning in health education requires access to a viable health education experience and equity in its delivery. It requires a commitment from schools to incorporate the most effective instruction and assessment. It requires teachers to be strategic planners who will engage and motivate students through seamless instruction to address personal health issues. "For effective learning to take place, students should be actively involved in the learning and be encouraged to use their particular skills/intelligences to demonstrate knowledge and skills."[15]

Learning requires a commitment from students to create quality work and strive for excellence; use a variety of learning strategies, personal skills, and time management skills to enhance learning; and reflect on and evaluate their learning for the purpose of improvement.[16] When students learn with understanding, they have a strong base for subsequent learning, which enables them to connect new knowledge to what they already know and gives them the capacity to refine skills for use in more complex settings.

The variety of learning styles requires differentiation in health instruction. Some learners need to absorb life experiences through their senses. They like to have a reason for learning new information or adapting new behaviors. They like to discuss. Others learn by analyzing data and drawing conclusions from them. Such students want to use facts to obtain a deeper understanding of what needs to be done and how to do it. Still others will want an opportunity for self-discovery; they want to feel the experience by interacting with others.[15]

Learning as it relates to health education is enhanced through parents and other significant adults when they communicate the value of health via modeling, reinforcing observed healthy behaviors, and collaborating with students on projects to enhance school/community health.

Adequate instructional time is necessary for learning to take place.[17] It is essential to master health education concepts and skills as outlined in the NHES grade span standards and indicators. After 10 years of implementation and assessment of the original NHES and examination of a variety of studies, it is recommended that students in Pre-K to grade 2 receive a minimum of 40 hours and students in grades 3 to 12 receive 80 hours of instruction in health education per academic year.

The importance of providing adequate instructional time in health education is recognized by both the public health and education communities. Healthy People 2010's Objective 7–2 focuses on the need to increase the number of middle/junior high and senior high schools that offer health education to lower the incidence of the following six risk factors: risky sexual behavior, intentional and unintentional injuries, tobacco use, alcohol and other drug use, poor nutrition, and physical inactivity.[18] The National School Boards Association has reported on research pertaining to the time necessary for effective health education. One study showed that 1.8 hours of health instruction per week over the school year produced measurable increases in student knowledge and improved attitudes about health; it also resulted in some behavioral changes. Another study demonstrated that health knowledge begins to increase after 15 hours of instruction, particularly in grades 4 to 7; 45 to 50 hours of instruction were needed to begin to affect attitudes and practices, with maximal learning and attitude or behavior changes occurring after about 60 hours of instruction in a given year.[19]

Learning is a joint effort. It requires from students the desire to learn. It requires that schools provide access to the possibility of learning and equity in the manner in which it is addressed. It requires time on task and authentic engagement to make it real enough that students value their health and transfer the knowledge and skills gained to personal application.

All the processes involved in understanding a concept take a great deal of time. Real, usable knowledge cannot be constructed from brief exposures to information.

—Lauren B. Resnick and Leopold Klopfer, *Toward the Thinking Curriculum: Current Cognitive Research*

The Essential Role of Partners in Implementing the National Health Education Standards

Teaching students to adopt health-enhancing behaviors requires a collaborative effort on the part of all who value the health and well-being of children. Educational agencies cannot do this alone. The adage "It takes a village to raise a child" could not be more appropriate than in raising a healthy child. Those sharing in this endeavor can take specific actions to encourage children to be healthy. Local education agencies (LEAs); state education agencies (SEAs); institutions of higher education (IHEs); national organizations and agencies (NOAs); community agencies, organizations, institutions, and businesses (CAOIBs); and families and caregivers have important roles involving access to and equity in the provision of health education for all children. The following section describes the essential action steps that each partner can take to address each of the Access and Equity Principles—Environment and Climate, Teaching, Curriculum, Assessment, Technology, and Learning—in the implementation and maintenance of a quality health education program.

Local Education Agencies

The essential role of the LEA is to provide administrative leadership and policy development in local schools to support the implementation of the NHES. District leaders, such as superintendents, principals, and curriculum coordinators, play an essential role in the ongoing development of effective school health education programs by being advocates for health education. Local education agencies can support the development and implementation of a pre-K–12 health education curriculum, provide professional development for teachers and school personnel, assist with continual improvement of curricula and programs based on data collection and analyses, and work with the community to establish a collaborative partnership for implementation of the NHES.

Supportive district and local policies and practices are vital to the success of effective school health curricula and programs. Examples of areas of support include a safe and healthy school environment, appropriate class sizes, adequate budgets and staffing, instructional time and resources to address diverse learning needs, and alignment of district health education policies with state policies, rules, and regulations.

Supportive district and local practices often include adoption of a theory-based health education curriculum taught by qualified health education teachers; the use of multiple assessment strategies in curriculum and instruction; the ongoing evaluation of health-related programs that serve students, teachers, and

Table 3.2 Local Education Agency Action Steps for Implementing the NHES

Access and Equity Principle	Action Steps
Environment and Climate	• Establish policies that provide a health-promoting environment that supports comprehensive school health education across all grades and buildings in a district. • Provide equitable space, class size, and access to facilities for school health instruction, comparable to that provided for other disciplines. • Provide a health education coordinator to facilitate pre-K–12 communications across multiple schools in a district. • Provide a school environment and classroom climate in which students and teachers feel comfortable, safe, and supported. • Encourage ongoing parent and community involvement in school health education programs.
Teaching	• Ensure that health education is taught by licensed/certified health education teachers. • Support teachers in planning, implementing, and aligning health instruction with the NHES and/or state standards. • Provide high-quality, ongoing professional development in health education content and pedagogy for teachers and school personnel. • Provide teachers with the time and financial resources that they need to meet the goals of the NHES.
Curriculum	• Establish policies and provide supervision and support to ensure that comprehensive health education is being implemented on the local level. • Implement a district-wide pre-K–12 comprehensive school health curriculum that is aligned with the NHES and/or state standards. • Administer the health education curriculum in a manner that is consistent with best practice recommendations from state and federal agencies and/or professional education and health organizations, e.g., it is research based, teacher supported, unbiased, gender sensitive, multicultural, and based on health needs and outcomes. • Update and revise the district-wide health education curriculum, in alignment with the NHES, on a regular revision cycle, with leadership from school principals and curriculum coordinators in collaboration with licensed/certified health educators.

(continued)

Table 3.2 (*continued*) Local Education Agency Action Steps for Implementing the NHES

Access and Equity Principle	Action Steps
Assessment	*Student Assessment* • Use authentic student assessments to determine whether the goals of the NHES and/or state standards are being met. • Require the reporting of student progress in health education. • Provide ongoing professional development in student assessment and curriculum evaluation to health education teachers. *Program Evaluation* • Collect data to show the effectiveness of the health education curriculum and its connection to academic achievement. • Use program evaluation to determine whether students are meeting the goals of the NHES and/or state standards. • Use student, staff, and program evaluations to determine whether funding is adequate to support and sustain quality health education instruction. • Use community assessments to determine awareness of and support for pre-K–12 comprehensive health education.
Technology	• Provide adequate access to technology, equipment, and resources for students, teachers, and school personnel in health education instruction and program development. • Provide training in how to effectively use technology in the delivery of health instruction to meet the goals of NHES.
Learning	• Require the implementation of a health education program of study for pre-K through grade 12 that is responsive to developmental levels and learning styles. • Schedule sufficient instructional time in health education for student acquisition of knowledge and skills, allowing for active participation in the learning process and giving opportunities to practice skills, reflect, problem solve, create new problems, and think.

school personnel; and the implementation of a school health advisory council to coordinate curriculum and program development, especially the implementation of the NHES.

The following are two examples of LEA leadership:

1. To make the connection between health and academics, an independent southeastern school district assesses students on their health-related skills as an indicator for school academic performance.
2. To create a win/win situation, a mid-Atlantic school district hires elementary health education specialists to deliver health education for students in kindergarten through fifth grade. Health education is scheduled during the school day and delivered by a certified health educator as a special-area subject, which allows for additional planning time for grade level teams.

Local educational agencies, working collaboratively with teachers, administrators, and school boards, can help implement the NHES through the action steps outlined in **Table 3.2**, which are organized by the six Access and Equity Principles.

State Education Agencies

The essential role of the SEA is to provide guidance and support to LEAs on state policies and guidelines and to offer assistance on the development of local policies, which includes implementation and assessment of the NHES. State education agencies, through collaboration with government agencies and businesses, acquire funding and resource opportunities to support local program efforts. Designating a health education leadership position within the SEA provides a point person for the acquisition and dissemination of current health knowledge and practices to LEAs. Through this leadership, the SEA provides direction, training, and technical assistance to administrators, teachers, school board members, and other interested professionals involved in the implementation of standards-based health instruction that is aligned with the NHES. State education agencies also play a supporting role in the creation, selection, and/or implementation of a sequential, pre-K–12 health education curriculum that provides students with the knowledge, skills, and attitudes to practice healthy behaviors.

The following are two examples of SEA leadership:

1. Making the connection with pre-service teachers, the health specialist in a Pacific Northwest state facilitates health education standards and assessment training each year for students at the university. The training

includes the use of best practices in health education, implementation of a standards-based classroom, and development and scoring of authentic student assessments. The specialist also facilitates two meetings a year with five to nine IHEs; agenda items include teacher certification, statewide professional development opportunities, undergraduate and graduate-level health education programs, updates on state content standards and new resources, and updates on coordinated school health sites and partnership opportunities.

2. Collecting data to improve health education, a southern state's coordinated school health program assessed the status of health education in its sixty-seven public school districts. An online needs assessment was sent to the comprehensive health education curriculum specialist in each district (LEA). The assessment included questions on curricula selection, use of certified health education teachers, the delivery of health education through integration or stand-alone courses, professional development needs, and local policy. Results were compiled and shared with district specialists and other partners. The data led to the development of a plan to strengthen and support local programs in the implementation of the state standards for health education, which were based on the NHES.

Working collaboratively with LEAs and other health education professionals, SEAs can help implement the NHES through the action steps shown in **Table 3.3**, organized by the six Access and Equity Principles.

Institutions of Higher Education

The essential role of an IHE is to prepare future health teachers (pre-service), classroom educators (in-service), and school leaders with the knowledge, skills, and competencies to promote adoption of the NHES in pre-K–12 curriculum, instruction, and assessment. An IHE must also require health education coursework for elementary education majors, who will be responsible for the delivery of health instruction within the school day. Within this context, it is expected that IHEs will prepare teacher candidates to meet the elementary, middle, and high school health education competencies outlined by national professional organizations and seek partnerships with LEAs and SEAs in their states to promote the use of NHES in pre-K–12 teacher training and curriculum deliberation. Institutions of higher education also need to maintain the professional development of their own faculty, expanding school health education understanding and competencies in the implementation and assessment of the NHES.

It is imperative that IHEs promote health education as essential coursework in pre-K–12 teacher licensure programs and as foundational preparation for

Table 3.3 State Education Agency Action Steps for Implementing the NHES

Access and Equity Principle	Action Steps
Environment and Climate	• Establish policies or regulations that identify health education as a required program of study and establish a climate for successful program implementation. • Support LEAs in the establishment of safe, nurturing school environments that are conducive to learning and model appropriate health practices.
Teaching	• Set professional standards for teacher licensure in health education in collaboration with accreditation agencies and institutions. • Ensure that high-quality professional learning, which includes work/study, collaboration, and professional development, occurs and is available for all teachers, curriculum specialists, and district leaders. • Ensure that high-quality professional learning is aligned with the SEA's professional standards for teaching practices and with professional learning as defined by the National Staff Development Council. • Provide statewide support to all teachers in the area of best practice for health education instruction. • Require that highly qualified teacher standards, stated in federal legislation, be applied to health educators. • Provide teacher training and professional development with a focus on standards-based instruction, including guidance to schools on periodic monitoring of compliance and quality control issues. • Promote differentiated instruction in professional development opportunities to meet the emotional, intellectual, physical, and social needs of all students.
Curriculum	• Employ appropriately certified/licensed school health educators and specialists within SEAs to provide leadership and assistance to local schools and communities. • Provide LEAs with the curricular and instructional support materials, such as state standards, scope and sequence, alignment and mapping tools, and frameworks, that are needed to meet the NHES and/or state standards. • Support LEAs by promoting pre-K–12 health education curricula and programs that are consistent with best practice recommendations of state and federal agencies and/or professional education and health organizations.

(continued)

Table 3.3 (continued) State Education Agency Action Steps for Implementing the NHES

Access and Equity Principle	Action Steps
Curriculum (continued)	• Where appropriate, guide LEAs to adopt research-based health education curricula and programs that are aligned with the NHES. • Provide support and technical assistance to LEAs in the area of data collection and analysis relative to health education curricular decisions. • Support cross-disciplinary articulation of health information and services through training, publications, and resources.
Assessment	• Provide LEAs with ongoing assessment training in NHES-aligned curricula so they can work with teachers and administrators to develop their own local assessments of students. • Provide support to districts in writing, developing, and scoring authentic student assessments to determine whether the goals of the NHES are being met. • Develop and implement a statewide assessment program that addresses health knowledge and skills across the pre-K–12 curriculum.
Technology	• Provide electronic resources with NHES-aligned, sample instructional and assessment activities to teachers across the state. • Implement and maintain a web site for health education that provides links, updates, registrations, and resources in the state. • Encourage and support schools through training and funding to use technology to extend and expand instructional capacity. • Ensure that pre-K–12 health education is part of the state and local technology plans. • Provide technology training and support for the delivery of NHES-aligned curriculum, instruction, and assessment. • Encourage local districts to adopt instructional materials that use diverse technology tools.
Learning	• Support the provision of adequate instructional time for the attainment of the NHES. • Provide training on differentiated learning. • Use student behavioral data, and the impact of those behaviors on learning, to support programs that enable students to reduce barriers to learning.

school administrators and health service professionals at the graduate level. Those who pursue a health education degree with teacher licensure should have access to accredited programs that promote the NHES in coursework and internships. The National Council for Accreditation of Teacher Education requires that all teacher candidates demonstrate their teaching impact on pre-K–12 student learning prior to graduation.

The following are two examples of IHE leadership:

1. Making health a priority, education majors at a southwestern university enroll in a Child and Adolescent Health course that addresses teacher health literacy. Pre-service education students are given opportunities to create instructional modules that address pediatric and adolescent health issues that incorporate the NHES for specifying learning strategies and performance outcomes. The course emphasizes evidence-based approaches for school health instruction and curriculum design and the teacher health education skills that maximize student health literacy through utilization of the child and adolescent health logic framework.[20]

2. Making interdisciplinary connections, a midwestern university health education faculty works across departmental lines to advocate and design health education courses to serve majors in early childhood education, middle childhood education, special education programs, and health education, resulting in a core of four pedagogy courses with a developmental aging perspective. These core courses focus on health issues of children and youth; teacher wellness; literacy and health; the relationships between curriculum, instruction, and assessment; coordination of education and health initiatives; and on using the NHES as a framework for curriculum design.[7] A local school, in partnership with the university, rewrote their health course of study so that it would be aligned with the NHES, adopted a comprehensive pre-K–12 school health curriculum, in-serviced teachers and health professionals in the new curriculum, established a health coordinating council, and hired a wellness coordinator within five years.

By working collaboratively with LEAs, SEAs, and other health education professionals, IHEs can help to implement the NHES through the action steps outlined in **Table 3.4**, as organized by the six Access and Equity Principles.

National Organizations and Agencies

National Organizations and Agencies affiliated with health and education are essential to the success of the NHES. They provide the professional guidance, administrative leadership, public policy development, and research that can and

Table 3.4 Institutions of Higher Education Action Steps for Implementing the NHES

Access and Equity Principle	Action Steps
Environment and Climate	• Address climate and environment and their relationship to learning in pre-service and in-service professional development opportunities. • Model an effective health education learning environment within higher education coursework.
Teaching	• Develop courses that enhance teacher health education skills and competencies through the NHES. • Prepare future teachers to use a variety of instructional methods, strategies, technologies, and resources in health instruction to meet the learning styles, interests, and needs of a diverse student population. • Encourage IHE administrators to provide support and incentives to health education faculty who lead in-service training in standards implementation and assessment through school/university/community partnerships. • Promote teaching and research opportunities related to the NHES and their assessment. • Expand the professional development of school health education faculty who promote the NHES in their teaching, research, and service commitments.
Curriculum	• Prepare future teachers to integrate health-related concepts with skills across the pre-K–12 curriculum, as guided by the NHES. • Advocate for NHES alignment in pre-K–12 curriculum development and deliberation at local, state, and national levels. • Promote the design, use, and dissemination of NHES-aligned, research-based curricula and programs in professional preparation coursework, internships, and fieldwork. • Influence faculty in health education, teacher education, educational leadership, and educational psychology programs to prepare future school professionals to use the NHES and to promote health as an essential element in academic achievement across the school curriculum.

(continued)

Table 3.4 (continued) Institutions of Higher Education Action Steps for Implementing the NHES

Access and Equity Principle	Action Steps
Assessment	• Prepare future teachers to create or select and use a variety of traditional and authentic assessments (e.g., portfolio and performance) to achieve the NHES. • Assist in pre-service and in-service workshops for teachers who need practice in assessing student work products in the context of their teaching practices and pedagogy. • Provide leadership in linking research to practice in school health education.
Technology	• Model the use of technology as a tool for curriculum, instruction, and assessment in professional coursework to support the effective and critical use of technology by future and current teachers.
Learning	• Assist in pre-service and in-service workshops for teachers who need support and experience with the synergistic effects of curriculum, instruction, and assessment. • Train teachers to use data to personalize, differentiate, and guide learning through the creation of a student-centered classroom. • Engage pre-service and in-service teachers in the development of skills to encourage and challenge students to succeed. • Encourage pre-service and in-service teachers to determine what is meaningful to students and use this knowledge for authentic engagement. • Prepare pre-service and in-service teachers to be student health education advocates, observing student progress and requesting all necessary instructional time and resources for learning mastery.

will support the implementation of the NHES and continuing improvements in comprehensive health education. High-quality health education is vital to the health profession as a discipline; therefore, professional organizations have a clear stake in this endeavor.

All NOAs concerned with health education for children and youth can help improve instruction through coordinated, collaborative efforts. The general public and all professionals in school health and public health need to be well informed about comprehensive school health education curricula and programs. The nature of undergraduate and graduate teacher education programs in colleges and universities is closely interwoven and related to pre-K–12 health instruction. Efforts to improve health education teaching and learning from pre-kindergarten through graduate education can be coordinated and supported by NOAs.

Policymakers at national, state, and local levels are in a unique position to view the broad range of influences on health education and to make decisions that promote improvements in the field. They can allocate funding and resources that are needed to study and implement improvements in health education. National organizations and agencies can also promote and examine teacher licensure standards and accreditation requirements to ensure that health education teachers have the rich background and content knowledge that are needed in the twenty-first century.

The following are two examples of NOA leadership:

1. Four national professional societies—the American Association for Health Education; the American School Health Association; the Society for Health, Physical Education, and Recreation; and the School Health Education and Services section of the American Public Health Association—formally agreed to participate in the development of the original 1995 NHES and the 2006 revision of the NHES. Financial support for the development of the standards was provided in collaboration with the American Cancer Society. These NOAs collaborated on a joint goal to advance pre-K–12 health education.
2. In a mid-Atlantic state, the American Cancer Society and the American Heart Association volunteered time and resources as part of a coalition that successfully advocated for health education leadership at the state level.

National organizations and agencies, working collaboratively with LEAs, SEAs, IHEs, and CAOIBs, can help implement the NHES through the action steps outlined in **Table 3.5**, as organized by the six Access and Equity Principles.

Table 3.5 National Organizations and Agencies Action Steps for Implementing the NHES

Access and Equity Principle	Action Steps
Environment and Climate	• Advocate for federal and state legislation that will help create safe and supportive environments for health instruction. • Protect and promote the health and well-being of children and youth. • Support and advocate for coordination of programs and services delivered in the school/community. • Advocate with policymakers at local, state, and national levels to ensure that all students, including those with special needs, have educational opportunities for pre-K–12 health instruction. • Partner with other education and health organizations to support policies related to pre-K–12 comprehensive school health education and NHES-based curricula, instruction, and assessments.
Teaching	• Support coalitions that bring together school health and public health educators for shared knowledge and action. • Provide high-quality professional development programs for LEAs, SEAs, and IHEs. • Support LEAs, SEAs, and IHEs in their efforts to provide professional development for teachers, faculty, administrators, and other health professionals who teach health in the schools. • Support and advocate for licensed/certified health teachers to teach pre-K–12 health education. • Support and advocate for quality pre-K–12 health instruction in public, private, and parochial schools. • Include health education concepts in national teacher examinations prior to licensure. • Assist in the development of quality measures and accreditation standards for health education programs.
Curriculum	• Employ professionally prepared health educators with curricular expertise within national health and education agencies and organizations. • Support state and local school systems in implementing NHES-based curricula, instruction, and assessments. • Work with partners to advance funding of comprehensive skills-based health education efforts, broadening categorical funding initiatives.

(continued)

Table 3.5 *(continued)* **National Organizations and Agencies Action Steps for Implementing the NHES**

Access and Equity Principle	Action Steps
Assessment	• Adopt polices that promote effective standards–based assessment practices in schools and universities. • Support research and evaluation efforts in schools, including ongoing assessment of: (1) student health skills and behaviors; (2) teacher knowledge, attitudes, and skills; and (3) parent and community interest and involvement in school health education. • Support LEAs and SEAs in their use of valid and reliable assessment tools when promoting NHES and/or state standards.
Technology	• Encourage innovative technology partnerships with IHEs and businesses. • Use advanced technology to educate health education professionals on the latest educational research and practices. • Develop quality measures and accreditation standards for electronic learning within the context of health education. • Advocate for unlimited access to computers and connectivity for pre-K–12 health education students and teachers. • Provide access, as available, for teacher training, parent and community education, and special programs.
Learning	• Provide high-quality professional development programs for teachers, faculty, and health professionals addressing effective student learning, e.g., understanding, applying, and transferring health skills and knowledge. • Provide current research and support materials focused on student learning to LEAs, SEAs, and IHEs for dissemination in pre-service and in-service health education efforts.

Community Agencies, Organizations, Institutions, and Businesses

The essential role of CAOIBs is to create partnerships that support the mission of schools in the implementation of the NHES. Ultimately, CAOIBs are interested in the development of a well-informed, healthy, and responsible citizenry.

Community agencies, organizations, institutions, and businesses include the following partners: health and social service agencies; school/community organizations and institutions; local government entities; faith-based organizations; print and broadcast media; and businesses and industry, including the organizations that represent them.

Although the missions of CAOIBs vary, those that focus on education and health are natural partners with local schools. For example, CAOIBs can play a key role in the sustainability of school health education through advocacy and participation as community partners. They can lobby for health and education legislation, adopt public policies advocating health education and health care for all children and their families, offer to fund incentive grants to support health education initiatives through school/community partnerships, provide specialized programs and training that focus on key health issues, provide academic service/learning experiences for pre-K–12 students, and purchase materials and equipment not funded by school budgets. They can also serve as representatives on school health advisory committees, healthy school teams, advisory committees, and curriculum councils.

The following is an example of CAOIB leadership:

In a midwestern school district, more than one hundred community representatives gave their time and talents toward crafting a common vision for the health and well-being of students in their school/community. To secure the understanding and support of the community's key decision makers, organizers invited prominent community and school leaders to a one-time school health advisory council meeting. Members interviewed key school administrators and community leaders to gather information about collaborative efforts within their school/community. As a result, the Public Education Network, based in Washington, D.C., funded the development of a three-year plan for health promotion and education in that district.

By working collaboratively with LEAs and other health education professionals, CAOIBs can help implement the NHES through the action steps outlined in **Table 3.6**, as organized by the six Access and Equity Principles.

Table 3.6 Community Agencies, Organizations, Institutions, and Businesses Action Steps for Implementing the NHES

Access and Equity Principle	Action Steps
Environment and Climate	• Support the adoption of a NHES-aligned curriculum for pre-K–12 health education as one component within a coordinated school health model. • Assist communities in offering accessible resources and needed health services that support the implementation of the NHES. • Provide funding for teacher training in overcoming language barriers and in translating materials that are sent home to support implementation of NHES.
Teaching	• Provide opportunities and incentives for training in teaching learner-centered health education classes based on the NHES. • Sponsor or support professional development for school staff, such as summer institutes or attendance at national conferences that promote the use of NHES. • Provide opportunities for teachers to work in health-related fields during the summer months and sabbaticals to enhance their health knowledge and skills.
Curriculum	• Participate with school personnel, students, and businesses or faith-based/cultural organizations to develop organized, planned, sequential health education curricula aligned with the NHES. • Advocate for all students to receive high-quality health education with a current curriculum that is aligned with the NHES. • Serve as community experts on curriculum development panels, review teams, and school health advisory groups.
Assessment	• Assist in mapping school/community resources and conducting a school/community needs assessment related to student achievement of the NHES. • Advocate for assessment and reporting of student progress in health education as an educational requirement.

(continued)

Table 3.6 *(continued)* **Community Agencies, Organizations, Institutions, and Businesses Action Steps for Implementing the NHES**

Access and Equity Principle	Action Steps
Technology	• Adopt/fund social marketing programs advocating NHES-aligned health education for all children and youth via electronic media and public service announcements. • Provide access to technology that schools may not have such as onsite conferencing, webcasting, and production of digital media to support and promote the use of the NHES.
Learning	• Provide resources such as facilities, guest speakers, and release time for employees to serve as volunteers in schools that would enhance the "real world" transference of NHES knowledge and skills. • Support varied classroom and community learning experiences that uphold the NHES.

Families and Caregivers

Families, especially parents and caregivers, are the primary health educators of children, youth, and young adults. A few adages seem appropriate in the context of health education: What is valued is modeled. What is known is taught. What is believed is acted upon. Most parents and caretakers want their children to be healthy and safe; to acquire the values, skills, and knowledge of a healthy life; and to be happy and productive contributors to society. With each generation, as more is known about health and the human condition, more responsibility falls on members of families to be vigilant about genetic, familial, and lifestyle health issues. The capacity to seek, question, and act on health information is invaluable to a family in its role of caring, protecting, and nurturing children, youth, and young adults.

The essential role of the family in the implementation of the NHES is as an active participant in and advocate for quality health education. Active participation includes becoming an educated voice—whether on local school health councils, school improvement teams, or other committees—in advocating for effective programs that are directed toward improvement of health

Access and
Equity Principles

behaviors. It includes becoming knowledgeable about health education, youth development, and current health issues that may affect their children and advocating for effective curricula, instructional time, certified teachers, and resources. It includes being informed about the health education program provided in their child's school, partnering with their child's health educator to teach and reinforce health skills, and leading by example, effectively modeling positive health practices for their children.

The following is an example of leadership by families and caregivers:

In a mid-Atlantic state, concerned parents initiated a campaign that was taken to the school board. This resulted in the implementation of middle school health education and increased physical education opportunities for students in the district.

Families, working collaboratively with LEAs and other health education professionals, can help implement the NHES through the action steps outlined in **Table 3.7**, as organized by the six Access and Equity Principles.

Table 3.7 Families and Caregivers Action Steps for Implementing the NHES

Access and Equity Principle	Action Steps
Environment and Climate	• Advocate for an instructional climate in which NHES-based instruction and assessment are valued components of the academic day. • Hold schools accountable for equitable class sizes, educational space, and instructional facilities for health instruction. • Attend parent-teacher conferences and school board meetings and inquire about the health instructional program. • Be an active participant in parent-teacher associations and organizations to support local school initiatives for health education of pre-K–12 students.
Teaching	• Request that teachers be licensed/certified to teach health education and to be held to the same standard of quality as teachers in other academic disciplines. • Request that health education teachers be required to engage in ongoing professional development. • Partner with pre-K–12 health educators in the delivery and support of health education skills and practices.

(continued)

Table 3.7 (continued) Families and Caregivers Action Steps for Implementing the NHES

Access and Equity Principle	Action Steps
	• Support health education teachers in the acquisition of educational resources needed to meet the goals of the NHES and/or state standards.
Curriculum	• Become informed about the local health education curriculum and its alignment with the NHES and/or state standards. • Advocate for and support a pre-K–12 comprehensive school health curriculum that is consistent with best teaching practices, is research based, and is differentiated for diverse types of learners. • Serve on health education curriculum teams, as appropriate.
Assessment	*Assessment* • Request that health education be assessed and included on the school report card. • Inquire about skill-based, authentic assessment practices in school health instruction. • Participate in student assessments that request parent and/or family involvement. • Discuss health instruction with children and monitor skill development and behavioral changes. *Program Evaluation* • Support the implementation of local or statewide assessments that give school districts data regarding the health behaviors of children and youth. • Request that the results of program evaluations be shared with local citizens to determine the ongoing needs for health instruction and program development.
Technology	• Advocate for equitable technology access and resources for pre-K–12 health education teachers and students. • Provide safe access to technology to support health education in the home, school, and community.
Learning	• Advocate for pre-K–12 health education as a required program of study, with specified instructional time, within state and local educational policies. • Advocate for an effective pre-K–12 health education curriculum that will provide optimal learning capacity and ongoing practice time for students. • Recognize and reinforce healthy behaviors exhibited by children and youth in the home.

References

1. Haycock, K., C. Gerald, S. Huang. 2001. Closing the gap: done in a decade. *Thinking K–16 (A publication of The Education Trust)*.

2. Schlechty, P. C. 2002. *Working on the Work. An Action Plan for Teachers, Principals, and Superintendents.* The Jossey-Bass Education Series. San Francisco, CA: Jossey-Bass (A Wiley Company), p.52.

3. U.S. Department of Health and Human Services. 2000. *Healthy People 2010, Volume I,* 2nd ed. Washington, D.C.: U.S. Government Printing Office. Available at http://www.health.gov/healthypeople/Publications

4. Gardner, H. 1999. *The Disciplined Mind: What All Students Should Understand.* New York: Simon & Schuster.

5. Jensen, E. 2005. *Teaching With the Brain in Mind,* 2nd ed. Alexandria, VA: Association for Supervision and Curriculum Development.

6. Tomlinson, C. 2003. *Fulfilling the Promise of the Differentiated Classroom: Strategies and Tools for Responsive Teaching.* Alexandria, VA: Association for Supervision and Curriculum Development.

7. Ubbes, V. A., T. L. Hall, and C. A. Falk. 2003. *Modules for Teaching & Learning About Health Education: A Study of Guiding Questions, Essential Readings, Critical Concepts, & Mental Models.* Mason, OH: Thomson Learning.

8. National Adolescent Health Information Center. 2005. *Improving the Health of Adolescents and Young Adults: A Guide for States and Communities.* Atlanta, GA: Centers for Disease Control, p. 8. Available at http://www.cdc.gov/HealthyYouth/Adolescent Health/Guide/order.htm/.

9. Florida Department of Education. 2005. *2005 Health Education Specifications for the 2006–2007 Florida State Adoption of Instructional Materials.* Available at http://www.firn.edu/doe/instmat/0607adoption/health_specs.pdf/.

10. Centers for Disease Control and Prevention. Division of Adolescent and School Health. Unpublished data available at http://www.cdc.gov/healthyyouth/

11. Centers for Disease Control and Prevention. 2005. *School Health Profiles 2005: Narrative Report.* Available at http://www.cdc.gov/HealthyYouth/profiles/2004/narrative.pdf

12. Marzano, R. J. 2000. *Transforming Classroom Grading.* Alexandria, VA: Association for Supervision and Curriculum Development.

13. Council of Chief State School Officers (CCSSO). 1999. *Assessing Health Literacy: A Guide to Portfolios.* CCSSO Health Education Project. Soquel, CA: Toucan Ed Publications, pp. 9–12.

14. Daggett, W. 2005. *International Center for Leadership in Education.* Presentation to Baltimore County (Maryland) Public Schools, High School Summit.

15. Anspaugh, D. J., and G. Ezell. 2001. *Teaching Today's Health,* 6th ed. Boston: Allyn and Bacon.

16. Seidel, K., and E. Short. 2005. Connecting students, standards, and success: using standards-based curriculum connections to improve learning. *Curriculum Leadership and Research Journal* 1:8.

17. Marzano, R. J. 2003. *What Works in Schools: Translating Research Into Action.* Alexandria, VA: ASCD.

18. U. S. Department of Health and Human Services, Centers for Disease Control and Prevention. 2000. Educational and community-based programs. In *Healthy People 2010, Volume I.* Washington, D.C.: U.S. Government Printing Office. Available at http://www.healthypeople.gov/document/html/volume1/07ed.htm

19. National School Boards Association. 1991, *School Health: Helping Children Learn.* Alexandria, VA: National School Board Association.

20. Peterson, F., R. Cooper, and J. Laird. 2001. Enhancing teacher health literacy in school health promotion: a vision for the new millennium. *Journal of School Health* 71:138–144.

4

Assessment

Measuring Excellence

When the chef tastes the soup, it's formative . . .
when the guest tastes the soup, it's summative.

—Robert Stake
Standards-Based and Response Evaluation

Overview

What should students be taught in the years between prekindergarten and grade 12? How can we determine whether students are learning what we want them to learn? And how do we determine whether the instructional strategies we are using actually succeed in helping students learn health education concepts and skills? Standards and assessment are valuable tools in answering these questions. Assessment serves a variety of purposes for teachers, students, administrators, other school personnel, family members, policy makers, business leaders, community members, and institutions of higher education.

The following section introduces assessment and assessment systems, identifies the purposes and principles of assessment, and discusses standards-based assessment, curricula, and instruction. It also describes the various types of assessment, identifies strategies for developing performance assessments, and provides examples of field-tested performance assessments in health education. This section also discusses professional preparation and development for assessment. A glossary of the terminology related to assessment can be found in Chapter 5, along with descriptions of resources and initiatives related to health education assessment.

Standards-based education is closely linked to assessment. Standards-based education demands clear identification of what students should know and be able to do. It is based on the assumption that the way to ensure that all students acquire specific knowledge and skills is to identify and teach to expected levels of performance for specific knowledge and skills. Standards should guide all decisions related to assessment, curriculum, and instruction, with the focus always on student learning.

For schools to be successful in achieving academic standards, it is essential for stakeholders in the schools, districts, and states to assess student learning, the instructional environment, and instructional programs. All individuals who are responsible for devising, administering, or overseeing the instructional program in the school must take a serious look at their role in guaranteeing that students are learning and making academic progress. The National Health Education Standards (NHES) identify the essential concepts that students should know and the essential skills students should have. Assessment provides the evidence by which it can be determined whether students have met the standards and performance indicators.

National and/or state standards and performance indicators are the foundation for assessment, curriculum, and instruction in health education. In a standards-based approach, assessments and assessment systems are aligned with standards and performance indicators. What we now know about learning indicates that assessment and learning are closely tied to each other. Because of this, it is important to clarify what we mean when we talk about assessment.

Clarifying Assessment

Assessment is a way to measure student learning. Assessment informs teachers and others what health-related concepts and skills students have learned, how well they have learned these concepts and skills, and whether or not adjustments must be made to health education curricula and/or instruction. *Assessment systems* combine multiple assessments into a comprehensive format that provides thorough, valid, reliable, and trustworthy information for making decisions about students' achievement. Assessment of student achievement of the health education standards and performance indicators is an important component of local and state assessment systems. Data regarding student understanding of health-related concepts and skills are critical to making informed decisions related to health education curriculum and instruction in classrooms, schools, districts, and states.

Assessments and assessment systems include formative or classroom-based assessments for learning and summative or high-stakes assessments of achievement. *Summative assessment* measures student performance based on established standards and criteria and usually leads to a report on student achievement or level of proficiency. *Formative assessment* continually measures student performance to guide instruction and enhance student learning. Emphasizing assessment *for* learning is perhaps more important than emphasizing assessment *of* learning because formative or classroom-based assessment can improve understanding of health-related concepts and skills and thus improve performance on summative or high-stakes assessments. An understanding of the purposes of summative and formative assessment is essential to making decisions related to assessment and assessment systems.

Purposes of Assessment

Summative and formative assessments serve many purposes in health education. Summative assessments, or assessments of learning, document student achievement of the state or national standards for health education.[1,2] Summative assessments, used in conjunction with formative assessments, can clarify the curriculum and instruction students will need to achieve the standards. Formative assessments, or assessments for learning, provide teachers and students with important information regarding students' understanding of health-related concepts and their ability to demonstrate health skills. Formative assessments give teachers information about the health-related learning needs of both individuals and groups of students. Formative assessments also supply teachers with timely feedback regarding the pacing of instruction and the need to re-teach and offer students additional opportunities to apply, practice, and master health-related concepts and skills. Formative assessments present students with important feedback related to their learning and ways to improve their work and achieve their learning goals.

Teachers use both formative and summative assessments to evaluate student learning, assign grades, and communicate with students and their families about student progress. Formative and summative assessments also provide important information for planning, implementing, and evaluating services and interventions designed to support student learning. Formative and summative assessments also guide professional development programs for teachers and other school personnel. Summative assessments ultimately verify student achievement of the NHES and the related performance indicators.

To select and administer quality assessments, a clearly defined purpose is essential. There are several important questions to consider when using an assessment:

- How will the results of the assessment be used?
  - To inform curriculum and instruction?
  - To assign a grade?
  - To document students' achievement of a standard and/or a performance indicator?
- What concept and/or skill is being assessed?
  - What level of knowledge of the concepts and/or ability to demonstrate health skill is being assessed: remembering, understanding, applying, analyzing, evaluating, or creating?
- What curriculum and instructional activities are needed to ensure that students have the opportunity to develop the knowledge and skill they need to succeed on the assessment?
- What resources are available for developing, conducting, and scoring the assessment and communicating the results of the assessment?

By answering these questions, teachers and other school personnel can decide the assessment activity or activities that best meet their needs. Another important question is: What are possible uses of assessment linked to NHES?

Uses of Assessment Linked to Standards

The NHES tied to assessment measures can be used for developing, refining, or evaluating assessment and assessment systems. For example—

- Teachers, curriculum directors, and other school personnel can use the standards to guide assessment reform in classrooms.
- Teachers, curriculum directors, and other school personnel can use the standards in their continuing professional development.
- Institutions of higher education, especially those involved in teacher preparation, can use the standards in their own instructional and assessment practices.
- Community, parent, advocacy, and business organizations can use the standards to evaluate and help improve student assessment systems.
- Policymakers who are developing new systems of assessment at the national, state, and district levels can use the standards to rethink the role of large-scale assessment and ensure support for classroom-based assessment.
- Educational researchers can use the standards to design, research, and conduct evaluations of schools and school systems.

The preceding section highlights uses of assessments linked to the NHES. In addition to considering the purposes and uses of an assessment, it is also important to keep in mind the guiding principles of assessment.

Guidelines for Assessment

The guidelines for assessment include:

- Promotion of learning.
- Alignment of standards, assessment, curriculum, and instruction.
- Use of multiple assessments that provide fair, valid, and reliable information about student learning.
- Clear and publicly communicated expectations, performance criteria, and assessment results.
- Regular review and improvement of assessment systems.

Guiding Principles of Assessment

There are key guidelines related to the appropriate development and use of assessment and assessment systems by classroom teachers, school administrators, and state and national policymakers. These key principles include the following:

- Promotion of student learning
- Alignment of standards, assessment, curriculum, and instruction
- Use of a variety of equitable, valid, and reliable assessments that ensure flexibility to meet the needs of a diverse student body
- Provision to students of clear information about performance criteria
- Provision to students of multiple opportunities to apply and master health-related concepts and skills and ongoing feedback to enhance their learning of these concepts and skills
- Provision to students and family members of information regarding student achievement
- Ongoing review and improvement of assessments and assessment systems

The preceding principles guide the appropriate use of assessment by classroom teachers, school administrators, and state and national policymakers.

Health education assessment is dynamic and continuous and does not occur in a vacuum. Assessment for learning in health education includes giving students explicit information about the health-related concepts and skills that will be covered by an assessment; clear performance targets prior to instruction; clear evaluation criteria; multiple models or demonstrations of excellence (*exemplars*); multiple opportunities to learn, practice, and apply health-related concepts and skills; assessments in which they create products and performances that are authentic in the application of health concepts and skills; support for assuming responsibility for learning; opportunities to engage in regular self-assessment; opportunities to build their confidence as learners; and frequent and specific feedback that gives them insight about ways to improve. Assessment for learning in health education also includes continual modification of instruction based on the results of classroom assessment and involvement of students in communication with their families about their progress toward, and achievement of, health literacy.[3,4]

The alignment of standards, assessments, curricula, and instruction is also important. For example, during a district-wide workshop, teachers, administrators, and other school personnel would determine which assessments would be appropriate to demonstrate proficiency in state or national standards for health education. When that is accomplished, staff would then design classroom instruction founded in theory-based curriculum to learn the skills needed to demonstrate standards and complete the assessments.

It is important for a teacher and other school personnel to use a variety of *equitable, valid,* and *reliable* assessments. Assessments that are equitable, valid, and reliable provide students with fair and legitimate opportunities to demonstrate their ability to achieve national or state health education standards. The use of a variety of assessments helps ensure flexibility in meeting the needs of a diverse student body.

Educators, schools, and districts should be providing students and family members with information regarding student achievement in health education. Assessment for learning in health education includes involving students in communication with their families about their progress toward and achievement of health literacy. For example, the health educator can communicate with parents to share a child's progress toward achievement of the NHES.

Finally, teachers should be reviewing and improving assessments and assessment systems on an ongoing basis to ensure alignment with state and national standards and curriculum. Requiring staff to update and align their health education assessments with the NHES during the five-year curriculum review process is one example.

The preceding guiding principles also apply to the development of assessment systems for health education. What is a comprehensive assessment for health education?

A Comprehensive Assessment System

A comprehensive assessment system for health education includes multiple tiers of assessment (classroom, school, district, and state). Comprehensive assessment systems inform and guide teaching and learning, establish accountability for monitoring and achieving standards, and certify the achievement of the standards.[5] Comprehensive assessment systems include both state and local data (**Fig. 4.1**).

The lowest tier (classroom, school, and district assessment) is where multiple authentic assessments can occur. Students are given the opportunity to demonstrate their skills and knowledge in ways that are meaningful. For example, a teacher may want to assess his or her students' knowledge and skills about the importance of wearing a helmet and how to wear a helmet correctly. The assessment may be a poster or a public service announcement regarding the importance of wearing a bicycle helmet, or a demonstration of the correct use of a bicycle helmet.

At the highest tier (state), an assessment of learning takes place. A state department of education, for example, can provide a comprehensive assessment system that includes both state testing and local assessment systems. In one state, local assessment systems are required to include at least 75% "common" assessments in each grade span.[6] These "common" assessments are assessments that all teachers at a specific grade level use for inclusion in the local education agency's assessment system.[6]

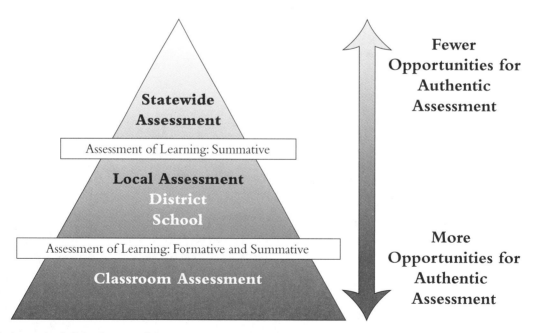

Figure 4.1 A standards-based comprehensive assessment system. It employs overlapping tiers of assessment (classroom, school, district, state) and aligns with standards, curricula, and instruction.

Adapted from the Maine Department of Education, *LAS Guide: Principles and Criteria for the Adoption of Local Assessment Systems,* 2004.

Standards-Based Assessment, Curriculum, and Instruction

We know that a guiding principle of assessment is the alignment of standards with assessment, curriculum, and instruction. The link between assessment, curriculum, and instruction can be thought of as a continuous cycle in which the assessment of standards and performance indicators informs curriculum, curriculum informs instruction, instruction informs assessment, and assessment once again informs curriculum (**Fig. 4.2**). Approaches to standards-based assessment, curriculum, and instruction include *backward design* and *curriculum mapping*. Additionally, the use of *universal design* helps ensure that standards-based assessment, curriculum, and instruction will accommodate the diverse needs of students.

Backward Design

Planning in a standards-based environment is often called "backward" because it "begins with the end" in mind.[7] In a standards-based classroom, "the end" that teachers concentrate on involves the standards and performance indicators that have been identified as those that students must meet at the end of the grade or course that they are in (versus completion of a particular activity or project, chapters in a book, or a packaged curriculum). Standards and performance indicators help clarify that what students are doing on a day-to-day basis

Approaches to Standards-Based Assessment, Curriculum, and Instruction

- The *backward design* model and *curriculum mapping* are used to align standards, assessment, curriculum, and instruction.

- *Universal design* is used to accommodate standards, assessment, curriculum, and instruction to the diverse needs of students.

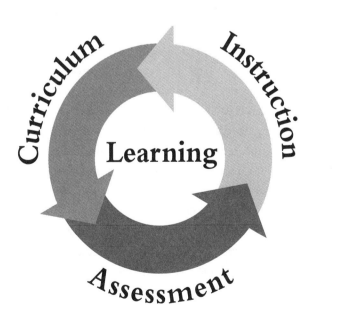

Figure 4.2 The continuous cycle of assessment, curriculum, and instruction, all of which inform each other.

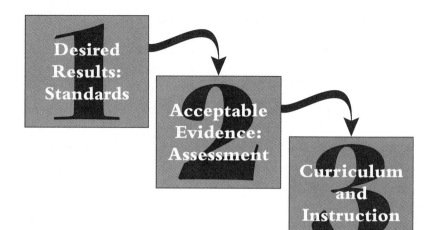

Figure 4.3 The backward-design approach to standards-based assessment, curriculum, and instruction. Standards arise from the desired results; assessment provides evidence that students are meeting or not meeting standards, which allows educators to shape curricula and instruction.[7]

Adapted, with permission, from Stages in backward design process. G. Wiggins and J. McTighe in *Understanding By Design, Expanded 2nd Edition, 2005.* Alexandria, VA: ASCD, 2005. Copyright © 2005 by Association for Supervision and Curriculum Development. Reprinted with permission.

is tied to the outcomes sought for the school year and for their entire pre-kindergarten–grade 12 educational experience. Assessments tied to standards and performance indicators provide clear pictures for students of the "end in mind" and provide direction for curriculum and instruction. Clarifying curricular priorities is another key component of backward design. Curriculum and assessment decisions are made based on the desired end result. The desired end result in health education is the set of health-related concepts and skills that students must know and be able to do to engage in healthy behaviors.

Backward design is a three-stage approach to aligning standards, assessment, curriculum, and instruction with a specific goal in mind[7] (**Fig. 4.3**). The first stage in backward design is to use standards and performance indicators to identify the health-related concepts and skills that students should know and be able to do. The second stage is to identify assessments that will provide evidence of students' achievement of these concepts and skills. The third stage is to identify the curriculum and instruction that will help students learn and master the health-related concepts and skills. Although these three stages outline an approach to the design of assessment, curriculum, and instruction, it is important to understand that these stages are interconnected and that there will be interplay between the development and implementation of assessments, curriculum, and instruction.

Backward design requires that teachers, administrators, and other school personnel make adjustments to teaching and learning in four key ways.[7] First, the assessments that are used to measure students' knowledge of health concepts and ability to perform health skills must be well thought out prior to the development of lessons. Second, favorite activities and projects may need to be revised or given up so that assessments will be in line with the NHES and performance indicators. Third, the methods and materials used for teaching health-related concepts and skills are chosen after teachers, administrators, and other school personnel have established the tasks that students must complete to demonstrate their knowledge and skills. Fourth, the resources used to support instruction in health education may shift from textbooks to a wide variety of materials, such as the Internet and information from governmental agencies (e.g., Centers for Disease Control and Prevention) and voluntary health organizations (e.g., the American Cancer Society).

Identification and development of assessments prior to the development of curriculum and instruction has many instructional dividends for teachers and students. It helps teachers more accurately analyze the health-related concepts and skills that are included in assessments, so that teachers can provide clear explanations of these concepts and skills. Selection of assessments prior to the development of curriculum and instruction also helps teachers to ensure that they include sufficient practice activities so that students have sufficient opportunities to learn and master health-related concepts and skills.[8]

Curriculum Mapping

Standards-based *curriculum mapping* also serves to align standards, assessment, curriculum, and instruction.[9–11] The first phase of curriculum mapping is the collection of data related to the concepts and skills currently being taught and the products and performances used to assess students' learning.[9] It is useful to integrate standards into the maps to determine the extent to which each standard is addressed through assessment, curriculum, and instruction.[8] This mapping of standards, assessments, curricula, and instruction provides information regarding the coverage and balance of assessment, curricula, and instruction with respect to each standard.

Universal Design of Instruction

Universal design of instruction is an approach used to maximize the learning of all students.[12] Universal design is the design of assessments, curriculum, and instruction so that they are usable by all students, to the greatest extent feasible, without the need for accommodations and adaptations.

Types of Assessment

- Assessment items vary according to the type of response requested of students.

- Assessment items lie on a continuum from informal assessment to formal assessment.

- Different types of assessment items are emphasized in formative assessment and summative assessment.

- The two major types of assessments include selected response items and constructed response items.

Assessment items vary according to the type of response that students are asked to provide by a question or prompt from a teacher. These assessment items lie on a continuum, from informal assessment (e.g., checks for understanding during classroom instruction) to formal assessment (e.g., questions on a statewide assessment). Further, different types of assessment items are emphasized in formative assessment (e.g., observation of students' ability to perform a skill during classroom instruction) and summative assessment (e.g., questions on a test).

The two major types of assessment items include *selected response items* and *constructed response items* (**Fig. 4.4**). Selected response items are questions in which the students are prompted to select an answer from two or more response options. Examples of selected response items include multiple choice, true/false, and matching items. Constructed response items are questions in which students are prompted to construct an answer to the question. Examples of constructed response items include fill-in-the-blank, short answer, essay, or other types of responses. Selected response and constructed response items are the types of items most commonly used on quizzes and tests to assess student understanding of health education concepts and skills. Constructed response items include

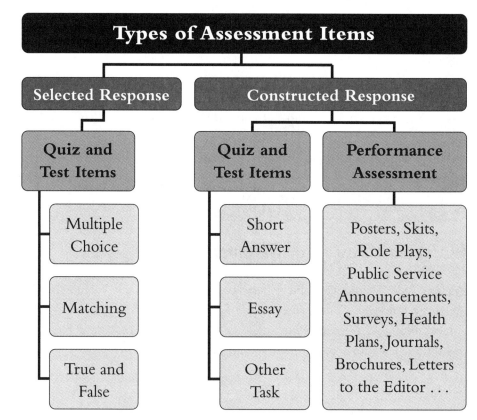

Figure 4.4 The different types of assessment.

performance events and *performance tasks.* Performance events and performance tasks are used for performance assessment.

Performance assessment is often referred to as *alternative assessment* or *authentic assessment.* Performance assessment requires students to create a product or performance which demonstrates their mastery of one or more health-related concepts and skills. These products or performances include, but are not limited to, exhibitions, investigations, demonstrations, skits, journals, and health plans (see **Fig. 4.4**). An "authentic assessment" generally refers to the real-life tasks and everyday situations that children and adolescents face. Therefore, a performance assessment in health education that is authentic will, for example, prompt students to write a letter to the school board to advocate for school breakfast; develop a script for refusing pressure to try a cigarette; or use the results of a self-assessment to make a personal health plan that includes short- and long-term goals for a healthy behavior, specific strategies to overcome barriers to the goals, sources of support, and strategies to monitor achievement of the goals.

Rubrics, Exemplars, and Anchor Papers

Rubrics, also known as *scoring guides,* inform student work in the development of performance assessments and teachers in the scoring of students' work. A typical rubric includes assessment criteria and a numeric (e.g., 4, 3, 2, 1) or linguistic (distinguished, proficient, apprentice, novice) scale designed to rate students' work. *Holistic rubrics* assess student work as a whole by assessing performance across multiple criteria. In contrast, *analytic rubrics* identify and assess the components of student work by assessing performance for each criterion. Refer to the section "Examples of Field-Tested Performance Assessments" for sample rubrics that accompany the three performance assessments included in this chapter.

Exemplars are prototypes or model samples of student work. Exemplars provide students with concrete examples of the products or performances they are expected to create or demonstrate. Exemplars also help teachers, students, and others evaluate completed student work.

Anchor papers are scored samples of student work that represent varying levels of achievement. Teachers use anchor papers to calibrate their scoring of student work.

Portfolios and Reflective Summaries

The products and performances that students create as a result of assessment are often included in portfolios. A *portfolio* is a representative collection of student work and is usually used to demonstrate student achievement over time. A *reflective summary* is a student-written explanation and evaluation of their work. Reflective summaries are often used in conjunction with formal performance events and with performance tasks. It is helpful to provide students with specific directions, a scoring rubric, and exemplars to guide them as they complete their reflective summaries.

A Continuum of Assessment

The types of assessment may be placed on a continuum of informal to formal assessment strategies (**Fig. 4.5**). At the informal end of this assessment are checks for understanding, whereas performance tasks fall at the formal end of this continuum. Classroom-based assessment embraces the full continuum of activities, whereas statewide testing is usually limited to selected response items. It is important to match the types of assessment used with the purpose of assessment.

Assessment Development

Assessment in health education includes the use of multiple and varying types of assessments. Ideally, these assessments will be matched to the intended use of the assessments and are equitable, valid, and reliable. Further, performance assessments are a wonderful vehicle to authentically assess students' understanding of health concepts and their ability to perform health skills.

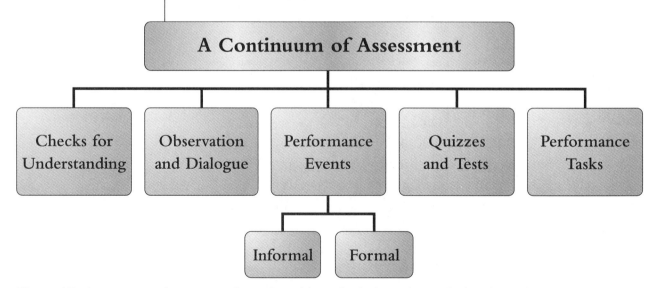

Figure 4.5 A continuum of assessment, from informal (e.g., checks for understanding) to formal (e.g., performance tasks).

Adapted, with permission, from A continuum of assessment. In G. Wiggins and J. McTighe: *Understanding By Design, Expanded 2nd Edition, 2005.* Alexandria, VA: ASCD, 2005. Copyright © 2005 by Association for Supervision and Curriculum Development. Reprinted with permission.

Validity and Reliability

A *valid* assessment is an assessment that measures what it is intended to measure (e.g., understanding of a specific concept or ability to perform a specific skill). To be valid, the assessment also needs to be reliable. An assessment is *reliable* when it is consistent in its measurement of a specific concept or skill.

Developing Performance Assessments

The components of a well-developed performance assessment include the following:

- A well-defined task that is aligned with one or two health education performance indicators
- A clear description of the task that provides—
  - Information about the concepts and skills the students will know and be able to do as a result of completing the task
  - A description of the product the student will create to demonstrate his or her understanding of the concepts and ability to perform the skill
- Step-by-step directions, including process steps, for receiving feedback and completing the task
- Assessment criteria, including the scoring rubric(s), and tips for a well-constructed task that will be used to assess the task
- The provision of exemplars
- Support for the task via specific instruction and opportunities for students to receive feedback and revise their work

Examples of Field-Tested Performance Assessments

The following pages contain three examples of field-tested performance assessments in health education, as well as the assessment tool, or scoring guide, that go with the prompt. These particular field-tested assessments were selected to demonstrate a variety of healthy topics, grade levels, or NHES, as well as three different resources (**Table 4.1**). All three assessments include the essential elements of a well-written assessment:

- Setting and role
- Goal or challenge
- Product performance
- Audience

The teacher will—

- Make it clear to the students what they need to know, understand, and be able to do and design projects that support the task
- Provide examples of excellent work
- Teach techniques and strategies to help students improve their performance
- Consistently check for student understanding
- Give clear, specific feedback to the students
- Adjust instruction, rubrics, and guidelines as needed to better meet the needs of the students
- Display student work to encourage and celebrate the achieving of the standard

The students will—

- Demonstrate a level of proficiency of the content areas
- Demonstrate a level of proficiency in skill development
- Self assess and make adjustments to their assignment/performance to better meet the requirements of the standard
- Monitor their grades and make adjustments to improve their achievement of the standard

Table 4.1
Examples of Field-Tested Performance Assessments

Grade Levels	NHES*	Topic	Name of Assessment
Pre-K–2 Example 4.1	Concepts and self-management	Injury Prevention	*Fire Safety*
6–8 Example 4.2	Concepts and advocacy	Nutrition	*Vending for Health*
9–12 Example 4.3	Concepts and accessing information	Alcohol, tobacco, and other drugs	*Tobacco Free Is the Way to Be*

*Assessment examples are based on the original 1995 NHES.

The Pre-K–2 assessment (**Example 4.1**) was written by the Council of Chief State School Officers (CCSSO), State Collaborative on Assessment and Student Standards (SCASS), and the Health Education Assessment Project (HEAP).[13] The assessment asks for students to design a map and key showing the floor plan of their home and yard and give a written description of the students' escape routes. Both concepts and self-management are the key standards to be assessed.

"Vending for Health" (**Example 4.2**) is a prompt for students in grades 6–8 developed by the Rocky Mountain Center for Health Promotion and Education.[14] Students play the role of a student council member who is challenged to write an article for the school newspaper advocating for the addition of juice and healthy snack machines. Students are scored using the Rocky Mountain Center's scoring guides in concepts and advocacy.

"Tobacco Free Is the Way to Be" (**Example 4.3**) is a high school prompt in which students design a brochure that includes advantages to being tobacco free as well as steps that former smokers may take to reduce their risk of using tobacco again. The product is scored by using both the concepts and accessing information scoring guides developed specifically for this assessment. This performance assessment was originally adapted from the SCASS Project for the Maine Department of Education.[15]

Performance Assessment

Injury Prevention—Fire Safety

 ## Topic

Every year many children die in house fires. Some of these fatalities could be prevented if fire escape options were discussed by families ahead of time. In this task, students will create personal maps that illustrate fire escape routes for their families.

Key Concepts

- risks of house fires
- importance of effective fire escape routes

Skills

SM—Self Management
- multiple escape routes identified
- family meeting place identified

Student Directions and Assessment Criteria

Project Description

Have you ever thought about what you would do if you woke up at night and realized that there was a fire in your home? Of course, you would want to get to safety as soon as possible!

Your Challenge

Your challenge is to develop a fire escape plan for your whole family. Since you will not know exactly where the fire may start, you will need to think about different escape routes for each room and a meeting place for your whole family once you are outside of the home. Use graph paper to draw a floor plan of your home and yard. Use colored pencils to show the routes for each room. Be sure to provide a key to your map, so it can be read easily. Then write a description of your plan, so your family will understand exactly what to do.

In your description, explain the importance of fire escape plans. Also describe the health risks of fires in the home.

Example 4.1 Pre-K–Grade 2 Assessment of "Injury Prevention—Fire Safety."

Reprinted, with permission, from the Council of Chief State School Officers (CCSSO), State Collaborative on Assessment and Student Standards (CCSSO-SCASS), Health Education Assessment Project (HEAP), 2005. Scored student work generated from this performance task is available through CCSSO-SCASS HEAP.

Performance Assessment

Project Options
Oral presentation

Demonstration

Assessment Criteria
You will be assessed on your ability to show concepts and skills that help you and others stay safe in a fire emergency. Your project must include a map and key showing the floor plan of your home and yard and a written description of your escape routes. Your written description must explain the importance of fire escape plans and the health risks of fires in the home.

KEY CONCEPTS
- risks of house fires
- importance of effective fire escape plans

SELF MANAGEMENT
- more than one escape route for each bedroom
- family meeting place

CCSSO-SCASS Health Education Scoring Rubric

CONCEPTS	SKILLS
4: The response is complex, accurate, and comprehensive, showing breadth and depth of information; relationships are described and conclusions drawn.	**4:** The response shows evidence of the ability to apply health skills; the response is complete and shows proficiency in the skill.
3: The response identifies relationships between two or more health concepts; there is some breadth of information, although there may be minor inaccuracies.	**3:** The response shows evidence of the ability to apply health skills; the response is mostly complete but may not be fully proficient.
2: The response presents some accurate information about the relationships between health concepts, but the response is incomplete and there are some inaccuracies.	**2:** The response shows some evidence of the ability to apply health skills. The response may have inaccuracies or be incomplete.
1: The response addresses the assigned task but provides little or no accurate information about the relationships between health concepts.	**1:** The response shows little or no evidence of the ability to apply health skills.

Example 4.1   (continued)

Performance Assessment

Vending for Health

Student Directions:

You are a student council member in your high school. In your student center there are vending machines selling a variety of snacks, such as soft drinks, chips, and candy bars.

Your challenge is to convince the school community to replace some of the current vending machines with ones selling juice, fruit, pretzels, and other healthy snacks.

You need to write an article for the school newspaper advocating for the addition of juice and healthy snacks machines.

You will need to convince other students, teachers, and administrators that this change will be beneficial for your school.

Answers will be scored on the following:

- How well you explain the negative health effects of soft drinks, chips, and candy

- How completely you explain the health benefits of juice, fruit and other healthy snacks

- How clearly you state a health-enhancing position supported by facts

---

Your article will receive a score on the Concepts standard and the Advocacy standard.

The rubrics on the back of this sheet will be used to score your article.

Example 4.2 Assessment of "Vending for Health."

Performance Assessment

Scoring Rubric for Concepts (CC)

NHES #1: Students will comprehend concepts related to health promotion and disease prevention to enhance health.

	Connections	Comprehensiveness
4	Completely and accurately describes relationships between behavior and health. Draws logical conclusion(s) about the connection between behavior and health.	Thoroughly covers health topic, showing both breadth (wide range of facts and ideas) and depth (details about facts and ideas). Response is completely accurate.
3	Describes relationships between behavior and health with some minor inaccuracies or omissions. Draws plausible conclusion(s) about the connection between behavior and health.	Mostly covers health topic, showing breadth and depth, but one or both less fully. Response is mostly accurate, but may have minor inaccuracies.
2	Description of relationship(s) between behavior and health is incomplete and/or contains significant inaccuracies. Attempts to draw a conclusion about the connection between behavior and health, but conclusion is incomplete or flawed.	Minimal coverage of health topic, showing some breadth but little or no depth. Response may show some inaccuracies.
1	Inaccurate or no description of relationship(s) between behavior and health. Inaccurate OR no conclusion drawn about the connection between behavior and health.	No coverage of health topic information. Little or no accurate information.

Scoring Rubric for Advocacy (AV)

NHES #8: Students will demonstrate the ability to advocate for personal, family, and community health.

	Health-Enhancing Position	Support for Position	Audience Awareness	Conviction
4	Extremely clear, health-enhancing position.	Thoroughly supports position using relevant and accurate facts, data, evidence.	Strong awareness of the target audience (e.g., the audience's perspective, interests, prior knowledge).	Displays strong and passionate conviction for position.
3	Generally clear, health-enhancing position.	Adequately supports position using facts, data, evidence; support may be incomplete and/or contain minor inaccuracies.	Adequate awareness of audience.	Displays conviction for position.
2	Unclear or conflicting positions.	Inadequately supports position, due to limited information, and/or some inaccuracy, irrelevant facts, data or evidence.	Some evidence of awareness of audience.	Displays minimal conviction for position.
1	No position stated OR position is not health-enhancing.	No accurate or relevant support for position is provided.	No evidence of audience awareness.	Conviction for position is not evident.

Example 4.2 (*continued*)

Performance Assessment

Tobacco Free Is the Way to Be

Student Page

Name: _____ **Date:** _____

In the U.S. hundreds of people die from smoking related diseases each year. Knowing how and where to get support to quit smoking will lower these statistics. Show what you have learned about staying or becoming tobacco free by creating a help brochure.

1. The self-designed brochure must contain:

   a. An analysis of 5 advantages of being tobacco-free. As part of the analysis, relate how being tobacco-free enhances an individual's well-being.
   b. List 4 steps a former tobacco user can take to reduce the risk of using tobacco again, including situations that should be avoided.

2. Complete the Resource Validity Form.

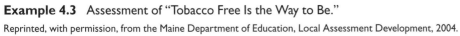

Example 4.3 Assessment of "Tobacco Free Is the Way to Be."

Reprinted, with permission, from the Maine Department of Education, Local Assessment Development, 2004.

Performance Assessment

Tobacco Free Is the Way to Be

Resource Validity Form

Name: _____

Date: _____

Directions:
1. List two products and three services that could help tobacco users quit.
2. Provide **evidence and a rationale (reasons)** verifying that each product or service is valid.

Title of Product/Service	Evidence and Rationale of Validity
1.	
2.	
3.	
4.	
5.	

Example 4.3 *(continued)*

Performance Assessment

Tobacco Free Is the Way to Be

Assessment Notes   **Revised 2/10/04**

Grade Span: 9–12

Assessment Type: Independent Design

Content (Topic) Area Groupings: Personal Health and Nutritional Health and Consumer Health, and Tobacco, Alcohol and Other Drug Use

Maine Learning Results: A1, B1
Standard A: Health Concepts
Students will understand health promotion and disease prevention concepts.
Performance Indicator:
1. Analyze the relationship between personal health practices and individual well-being.
Standard B: Health Information, Services, and Products
Students will know how to acquire valid information about health issues, services, and products.
Performance Indicator:
1. Provide evidence to support the validity of health information, products, and services.

Assessment Summary:
This task asks students to demonstrate their understanding of the advantages of being tobacco-free and to analyze the relationship between personal health practices and individual well-being. Students will evaluate types of products and services designed to help people resist or quit using tobacco and provide evidence on the Resource Validity Sheet that they are valid. Students will design a brochure containing an analysis of 5 advantages of being tobacco-free and how being tobacco-free enhances an individual's well-being and four steps a former tobacco user can take to reduce the risk of using tobacco again.

Review scoring guide with students.

Materials and Resources:
- Pens/pencils/paper/magazine pictures/computer
- Library/Internet for resource

Suggested Time Frame:
Two class periods of 45 min. each or one 90 min. block

Suggestions for Prior Instruction:
- Addictive properties of tobacco
- Health risks of tobacco
- Benefits of being tobacco-free
- Criteria for determining validity of resources, products and services
- Health products/services available for tobacco use cessation

Source of Original Assessment: Health Education SCASS II

Example 4.3 *(continued)*

Performance Assessment

Tobacco Free Is the Way to Be

Scoring Guide   **9–12 Health Education**

Content Standards and Performance Indicators	**1** attempted demonstration (does not meet standards)	**2** partial demonstration (partially meets standards)	**3** proficient demonstration (meets the standards)	**4** sophisticated demonstration (exceeds standards)
A. Health Concepts I. Analyze the relationship between personal health practices and individual well-being. Source of Evidence: Brochure	Brochure attempts to analyze the relationships between being tobacco-free and one's well-being and list examples of the advantages of being tobacco-free.	Brochure analyzes some of the relationships between being tobacco-free and one's well-being and provides some examples of the advantages of being tobacco-free.	Brochure accurately analyzes 5 advantages showing the relationships between being tobacco-free and one's well-being.	Brochure accurately analyzes in-depth 5 advantages showing the relationships between being tobacco-free and one's well-being.
B. Health Information, Services and Products I. Provide evidence to support the validity of health information, products, and services. Source of Evidence: Resource Validity Form	Student "Resource Validity Form" is incomplete or completed with significant errors.	Student accurately completes **most** of the "Resource Validity Form." Some evidence to support validity of products or services may be missing or inaccurate.	Student accurately completes the "Resource Validity Form" and clearly explains evidence to support validity for 4–5 products and services.	Student accurately completes the "Resource Validity Form" and clearly explains evidence and a rationale that verifies reliability for each product and service.

NS is considered a score and is assigned to student work for one of the following reasons:
- No evidence is available—no response, blank
- Student work is illegible
- Student work is completely off task

Example 4.3 (*continued*)

Professional Preparation and Development Related to Assessment

Teachers, principals, and other school personnel must have assessment-related knowledge and skills to effectively develop, implement, and evaluate student assessments in health education. Therefore, teachers, principals, and other school personnel need professional preparation and development to learn to develop or select appropriate valid and reliable assessments, as well as accurately and consistently score student work. Additionally, licensing standards must require that teachers, principals, and other school personnel be competent in assessment.

Professional preparation programs must enable pre-service teachers, administrators, and other school personnel to develop assessment-related knowledge and skills. Faculty at institutions of higher education can help pre-service teachers develop assessment-related knowledge and skills in the following ways: by modeling best practices in assessment as they assess future teachers' achievement in health education courses; by ensuring that pre-service teachers have an understanding of basic concepts (e.g., types of assessment) and principles (e.g., backward design) related to assessment in health; by providing future teachers with multiple opportunities to develop and administer different types of assessments to students in field experiences and evaluate the results of these assessments; and by providing pre-service teachers with resources to further develop their assessment-related knowledge and skills. Personnel at institutions of higher education must also provide future administrators with opportunities to develop knowledge and skills related to leadership in—and supervision of—assessment.

In-service teachers, principals, and other school staff also need professional development experiences to develop assessment-related knowledge and skills. Personnel at institutions of higher education, state departments of education, professional organizations, and school districts can help in-service teachers, administrators, and other school personnel develop assessment-related knowledge and skills by sponsoring professional development workshops, conference sessions, and online and face-to-face courses related to assessment in health education. They can also provide teachers, principals, and other school personnel with technical assistance and resources for health education assessment.

Summary

Assessment linked to health education standards, performance indicators, curriculum, and instruction is critical to students' mastery of health concepts and skills. Summative or high-stakes assessment of learning provides valuable

Professional Preparation and Development for Assessment in Health Education

- Teachers, principals, and other school personnel need pre-service professional preparation and in-service professional development to learn to effectively and efficiently plan, implement, and evaluate assessment activities in health education.

- State licensing standards must require teachers, principals, and other school personnel to be competent in assessment.

- Institutions of higher education must provide professional preparation experiences related to assessment. They must also collaborate with local and state education agencies and state and national health education organizations to provide professional development experiences related to assessment in health education.

The principles of assessment provide important guidance related to the appropriate use of assessment by classroom teachers, school administrators, and state and national policy makers.

The principles of assessment include:

- The promotion of learning

- The use of multiple sources of information

- The use of assessments that provide fair, valid, and reliable information

information about students' mastery of health concepts and skills, whereas formative or classroom-based assessment for learning is a valuable tool for enabling students to master these health concepts and skills. Assessment in health education serves a variety of purposes and provides important information for making decisions for students, schools, districts, and states. Principles of assessment include the promotion of learning; alignment of health education standards, assessment, curriculum, and instruction; the use of multiple assessments that provide fair, valid, and reliable information; clear and publicly communicated expectations, performance criteria, and assessment results; and regular review and improvement of health education assessments and assessment systems. Standards-based assessment in health education uses tiers of assessment at the classroom, school, district, and state levels. Backward design can be used to align standards, assessment, curriculum, and instruction. Universal design can be used to accommodate standards, assessment, curriculum, and instruction to the diverse needs of students.

There are a variety of types of assessment; these types of assessment fall on a continuum of assessment, from checks for understanding to performance tasks. The use of various types of assessment should be matched to the purpose of the assessment (assessment for learning and assessment of learning). Additionally, there are many valuable resources for supporting both the assessment of learning and the assessment for learning in health education. Further, pre-service professional preparation and in-service professional development for teachers, administrators, and other school personnel is critical to the effective use of assessment in comprehensive school health education.

References

1. Kolbe, L. J. 2002. Education reform and the goals of modern school health programs. *The State Education Standard* 3: 4–11.

2. Lohrmann, D. K., and Wooley, S. F. 1998. Comprehensive school health education. In *Health Is Academic: A Guide to Coordinated School Health Programs,* ed. E. Marx, S. F. Wooley, and D. Northrup. New York: Teachers College Press, pp. 43–66.

3. McTighe, J. 1996/1997. What happens between assessments? *Educational Leadership* 54: 6–12.

4. Stiggins, R. 2002. Assessment crisis: The absence of assessment for learning. *Phi Delta Kappan* 83: 758–765.

5. Maine Department of Education. 2004. LAS Guide: *Principles and Criteria for the Adoption of the Local*

Assessment System. Augusta, ME: Maine Department of Education.

6. Maine Department of Education. 2004. *Considering Consistency: Conceptual and Procedural Guidance for Reliability in a Local Assessment System.* Augusta, ME: Maine Department of Education.

7. Wiggins, G., and J. McTighe. 2005. *Understanding By Design,* Expanded 2nd ed. Alexandria, VA: Association for Supervision and Curriculum Development.

8. Popham, W. J. 2003. *Test Better, Teach Better: The Instructional Role of Assessment.* Alexandria, VA: Association for Supervision and Curriculum Development.

9. Carr, J. F., and D. E. Harris. 2001. *Succeeding With*

Standards: Linking Curriculum, Assessment, and Action Planning. Alexandria, VA: Association for Supervision and Curriculum Development.

10. Jacobs, H. H. 1997. *Mapping the Big Picture: Integrating Curriculum & Assessment K–12.* Alexandria, VA: Association for Supervision and Curriculum Development.

11. Jacobs, H. H. 2004. Development of a prologue: Setting the stage for curriculum mapping. In *Getting Results with Curriculum Mapping,* ed. H. H. Jacobs. Alexandria, VA: Association for Supervision and Curriculum Development, pp. 1–9.

12. Burgstahler, S. 2002. *Universal Design of Instruction.* http://www.washington.edu/doit/Brochures/ Academics/instruction.html.

13. Council of Chief State School Officers. 2004. Performance task: Injury prevention—fire safety. In *Assessing Health Literacy: Assessment Tools for Elementary Teachers,* 2nd ed. Washington, D.C.: CCSSO.

14. Rocky Mountain Center for Health Promotion and Education. 2005. *Vending for Health.* Lakewood, CO: Rocky Mountain Center for Health Promotion and Education.

15. Maine Department of Education. 2005. *Tobacco Free Is the Way to Be.* http://mainegovimages.informe .org/education/lsalt/LAD/Tasks/Health9-12/ TobaccoFree.pdf

Recommended Reading List on Assessment

Black, P., and D. Wiliam. 1998. Assessment and classroom learning. *Assessment in Education: Principles, Policy, & Practice* 5: 7–74.

Black, P., and D. Wiliam. 1998. Inside the black box: Raising standards through classroom assessment. *Phi Delta Kappan.* http://www.pdkintl.org/kappan/ kbla9810.htm

Council of Chief State School Officers. 1997. *Assessing Health Literacy: A Guide to Portfolios.* Washington, D.C.: Council of Chief State School Officers.

Council of Chief State School Officers. 2004. *Assessing Health Literacy: Assessment Tools for Elementary Teachers,* 2nd ed. Washington, D.C.: Council of Chief State School Officers.

Council of Chief State School Officers. 2004. *Assessing Health Literacy: Assessment Tools for High School Teachers,* 2nd ed. Washington, D.C.: Council of Chief State School Officers.

Council of Chief State School Officers. 2004. *Assessing Health Literacy: Assessment Tools for Middle School Teachers,* 2nd ed. Washington, D.C.: Council of Chief State School Officers.

Council of Chief State School Officers. 2004. *Fact Sheet: What Are the Differences Between Selected Response and Performance-Based Items?* http://www.ccsso.org/ content/pdfs/SCASSHEAPDifferencesSRandPB.pdf.

Council of Chief State School Officers. 2004. *Fact Sheet: What Is the Health Education Assessment Project?* http://www.ccsso.org/content/pdfs/SCASSHEAP Description.pdf.

Council of Chief State School Officers. 2004. *Fact Sheet: Your Guide to the CCSSO~SCASS HEAP Terms* http://www.ccsso.org/content/pdfs/SCASSHEAP terms.pdf

Marzano, R. J. 2000. *Transforming Classroom Grading.* Alexandria, VA: Association for Supervision and Curriculum Development.

McTighe, J. 2001. Assessing student learning in the classroom: Part II. *Health Educator* 1: 1–7. http://www .rmc.org/pdf/RMCHEV1N3BW.pdf.

McTighe, J. 2000–2001. Assessing student learning in the classroom-Part 1. *Health Educator* 1: 1–7. http://www .rmc.org/pdf/RMCHEV1N2BW.pdf.

McTighe, J., and G. Wiggins. 2004. *Understanding by Design Professional Development Workbook.* Alexandria, VA: Association for Supervision and Curriculum Development.

National Forum on Assessment. 1995. *Principles and Indicators for Student Assessment Systems.* Cambridge, MA: The National Center for Fair & Open Testing. http://www.fairtest.org/facts/principles%20PDF.pdf.

Northwest Regional Educational Laboratory. 1998. *Improving Classroom Assessment: A Toolkit for Professional Developers. Toolkit98.* http://www.nwrel.org/assessment/toolkit98.php.

Pateman, B. 2003/2004. Healthier students, better learners. *Educational Leadership* 61: 70–74.

Popham, W. J. 2004. Why assessment illiteracy is professional suicide. *Educational Leadership* 62: 82–83.

Popham, W. J. 2005. Instructional quality: collecting credible evidence. *Educational Leadership* 62: 80–81.

Popham, W. J. 2005. Students' attitudes count. *Educational Leadership* 62: 84.

Reeves, D. B. 2004. *Accountability for Learning: How Teachers and School Leaders Can Take Charge.* Alexandria, VA: Association for Supervision and Curriculum Development.

Rolheiser, C., B. Bower, and L. Stevahn. 2000. *The Portfolio Organizer: Succeeding With Portfolios in Your Classroom.* Alexandria, VA: Association for Supervision and Curriculum Development.

Safer, N. and S. Fleischman. 2005. How student progress monitoring improves instruction. *Educational Leadership* 62: 81–83.

Schmoker, M. J., and R. J. Marzano. 2003. Realizing the promise of standards-based education. In *Contemporary Issues in Curriculum,* ed. A. C. Ornstein, L. S. Behar-Horenstein, and E. F. Pajak. 3rd ed. New York: Allyn and Bacon, pp. 262–267.

Stiggins, R. 2001. The unfulfilled promise of classroom assessment. *Educational Measurement: Issues and Practice* 20: 5–15.

Stiggins, R. 2003. Assessment, student confidence, and school success. In *Contemporary Issues in Curriculum,* ed. A. C. Ornstein, L. S. Behar-Horenstein, and E. F. Pajak. 3rd ed. New York: Allyn and Bacon, pp. 197–207.

Strong, R. W., H. F. Silver, and M. J. Perini. 2001. *Teaching What Matters Most: Standards and Strategies for Raising Student Achievement.* Alexandria, VA: Association for Supervision and Curriculum Development.

5

Background on Standards Development

A Background for Excellence

Successful learners are not only knowledgeable and productive
but also emotionally and physically healthy, motivated, civically engaged,
prepared for work and economic self-sufficiency, and ready
for the world beyond their own borders.

—Health and Learning, ASCD 2004 Adopted Positions

Review and Revision Process

In June 1993, with support from the American Cancer Society, The Joint Committee for National Health Education Standards was formed with members from the American Association for Health Education (AAHE—formerly the Association for the Advancement of Health Education), the American Public Health Association (APHA), the American School Health Association (ASHA), and the Society of State Directors of Health, Physical Education, and Recreation (SSDHPER). Over the next two years, the Joint Commission underwent the process of developing the first National Health Education Standards (NHES). In 1995 the NHES were published, and over the following ten years, well over 200,000 copies were distributed, influencing 38 states to adopt or adapt the NHES for their use. In addition, several million dollars in federal and state funds had been dispersed in that time period to assist in the implemention and assessment of the standards. The impact of the NHES is seen in policy and program changes at national, state, and local levels. State adoption of the NHES often required legislative changes that heightened the awareness and importance of health education. In addition, all major health education curricula now reference the NHES.

In 2003, discussion began between the AAHE and the American Cancer Society (ACS), resulting in a proposal requesting funds to support a ten-year review and revision of the Standards. The ACS agreed to provide funding and staff support for the review, revision, and production of the revised NHES.

Committee Structure to Review and Revise the Standards

In summer 2004, a nomination process was announced to identify and select candidates to serve on the 10-Year Review and Revision Panel. Nominees were asked to submit letters of interest, identifying their past use and application of the NHES, as well as the expertise they would bring to the review and revision process. By early fall 2004, panel members had been selected, and in late September the panel held their first organizational meeting in Atlanta, Georgia. The eighteen-member panel included representatives from the national health education organizations involved in the development of the original NHES, as well as individuals representing K–12 health instruction, school health coordination, state departments of education, and institutions of higher education.

The charge to the panel members included the following components:

- Obtain and evaluate data regarding utilization of the 1995 NHES.
- Obtain and evaluate data regarding the perceived quality and usability of the 1995 standards, including strengths and weaknesses.

- Obtain and evaluate data regarding the assessments being used to evaluate progress on the 1995 standards at state and local levels.
- Examine current and future trends in education and health that may have relevance to the revisions needed.
- Review and revise the standards and performance indicators in light of the feedback obtained; this will include a discussion of how topical content areas will be addressed.
- Examine the translation of the 1995 NHES that occurred following their release, with particular emphasis on Standard 1, to determine whether "concepts" remain a valid need. If so, how can the standards be revised to reflect those concepts?
- Review and expand the opportunity to learn standards and incorporate guidance for the opportunity to learn standards as a focus of implementation strategies.
- Provide guidance on appropriate student assessment, including performance-based strategies and direction for assessment resources.

Building Consensus in Review and Revision

Over the next eighteen months, panel members were engaged in an active process to examine the current NHES, make recommendations for revision or restructuring, and develop related document sections and supportive materials to enhance use of the revised NHES. Each panel member served in two of six workgroups:

- Survey and Review
- Standards and Performance Indicators
- Introduction (Assumptions, Parameters, Definitions)
- Opportunity to Learn Standards (later changed to "Equity and Access")
- Guidance on Assessment
- Documents Review

Initially, comments were solicited from health and education professionals to gain an understanding of issues and challenges with the existing Standards. As the Standard Statements and Performance Indicators were revised, there were three online opportunities for professional review. Each time, responses were collected and thoughtfully reviewed as subsequent drafts were developed. The panel reviewed a variety of relevant resources and a number of NHES documents, including those from other educational disciplines and a number of states, to assess content, structure, and format as the new Standards document emerged. A final draft was sent to a few select reviewers for additional feedback prior to completion and pre-production editing.

John Whitehead said that "Children are the living message we send to a time we will not see." What kind of message will we send? We share a common desire to send children healthy and happy into their future. Let's redouble our commitment to give them the tools they need and will one day use when we are gone.

—Richard H. Carmona, MD, MPH, FACS, United States Attorney General

National Health Education Standards
Review and Revision Timeline

2004

May	• Call for nominations for Review and Revision Panel
July	• Review of panel member nominations/letters of interest
August	• Selection of panel members
	• Development of charge to panel
September	• First organizational meeting of NHES Review and Revision Panel, Atlanta, GA
October	• Identification of six small workgroups membership
	• Development of small workgroup assignments/charge
	• Gather field input on Standards use, assessment, and status
Oct–Dec	• Small workgroup conference calls
December	• Information/discussion forum on NHES Review and Revision at the CDC/DASH Funded Partners Meeting

2005

Jan–Feb	• Small workgroup conference calls
March	• Full NHES Review and Revision Panel Meeting, Atlanta, GA
April	• Small workgroup conference calls
	• First draft of Standards revision available online for public and professional review and comment
May	• Small workgroup conference calls
	• Full NHES panel conference call to review online survey results
June	• Small workgroup conference calls
	• Abstract presentation, IUPHE Conference, Stockholm, Sweden
	• Standards/PI small workgroup meeting
	• Full NHES panel conference call to review draft from Standards/Performance Indicators (PI)
	• Workgroup drafts of Standards/PI
July	• Final proposed Standards statements and 2nd draft of revised (proposed) PI online for public review
August	• Public review data gathered; summary sent to panel
	• Standards and PI workgroup meets to incorporate online comments
	• Full panel conference call
September	• All workgroup drafts to full panel for review
	• Full panel meeting—review and discussion of draft
Oct–Dec	• Workgroup drafts circulated to full panel for review; weekly conference calls to discuss and offer feedback

2006

January	• Small writing team assembled to finalize draft
February	• Final draft sent to select school health professionals for review
March	• Final draft completed—sent to ACS for editing, design, and production
April–Sept	• Production
Fall 2006	• Release of National Health Education Standards

Glossary

Achievement Tests

"Tests used to measure how much a student has learned in various school subjects. . . These norm-referenced, multiple-choice tests are intended to measure students' achievement in the basic subjects found in most school districts' curriculum and textbooks. Results are used to compare the scores of individual students and schools with others—those in the area, across the state, and throughout the United States." (Association for Supervision and Curriculum Development)

Alignment

"The process of linking content and performance standards to assessment, instruction, and learning in classrooms. One typical alignment strategy is the step-by-step development of (a) content standards, (b) performance standards, (c) assessments, and (d) instruction for classroom learning." (National Center for Research on Evaluation, Standards, and Student Testing, 1999)

Alternative Assessment (also Authentic or Performance Assessment)

"An assessment that requires students to generate a response to a question rather than choose from a set of responses provided to them. Exhibitions, investigations, demonstrations, written or oral responses, journals, and portfolios are examples of the assessment alternatives we think of when we use the term 'alternative assessment.' Ideally, alternative assessment requires students to actively accomplish complex and significant tasks, while bringing to bear prior knowledge, recent learning, and relevant skills to solve realistic or authentic problems. Alternative assessments are usually one key element of an assessment system." (National Center for Research on Evaluation, Standards, and Student Testing, 1999)

Analytic Scoring

"Evaluating student work across multiple dimensions of performance rather than from an overall impression (holistic scoring). In analytic scoring, individual scores for each dimension are scored and reported." (National Center for Research on Evaluation, Standards, and Student Testing, 1999)

Anchor(s)

"A sample of student work that exemplifies a specific level of performance. Raters use anchors to score student work, usually comparing the student performance to the anchor. For example, if student work was being scored on a scale of 1 to 5, there would typically be anchors (previously scored student work) exemplifying each point on the scale." (National Center for Research on Evaluation, Standards, and Student Testing, 1999)

Assessment

"The process of gathering, describing, or quantifying information about performance." (National Center for Research on Evaluation, Standards, and Student Testing, 1999)

Assessment System

"The combination of multiple assessments into a comprehensive reporting format that produces comprehensive, credible, dependable information upon which important decisions can be made about students, schools, districts, or states. An assessment system may consist of a norm-referenced or criterion-referenced assessment, an alternative assessment system, and classroom assessments." (National Center for Research on Evaluation, Standards, and Student Testing, 1999)

Authentic Assessment

"Assessment that measures realistically the knowledge and skills needed for success in adult life. The term is often used as the equivalent of performance assessment, which, rather than asking students to choose a response to a multiple-choice test item, involves having students perform a task, such as . . . writing a letter to the city council to advocate for spaces and facilities for physical activity . . ." (Association for Supervision and Curriculum Development)

Benchmark

"A detailed description of a specific level of student performance expected of students at particular ages, grades, or development levels. Benchmarks are often represented by samples of student work. A set of benchmarks can be used as 'checkpoints' to monitor progress toward meeting performance goals within and across grade levels." (National Center for Research on Evaluation, Standards, and Student Testing, 1999)

Classroom Assessment

"An assessment developed, administered, and scored by a teacher or set of teachers with the purpose of evaluating individual or classroom student performance on a topic. Classroom assessments may be aligned into an assessment system that includes alternative assessments and either a norm-referenced or a criterion-referenced assessment. Ideally, the results of a classroom assessment are used to inform and influence instruction that helps students reach high standards." (National Center for Research on Evaluation, Standards, and Student Testing, 1999)

Comprehensive School Health Education

The part of the coordinated school health program that includes the development, delivery, and evaluation of planned, sequential, and developmentally appropriate instructions, learning experiences, and other activities designed to protect, promote, and enhance the health literacy, attitudes, skills, and well-being of students from pre-kindergarten through grade 12. The content is derived from the National Health Education Standards and guidelines that are available in some states.

Coordinated School Health Program

An organized set of policies, procedures, and activities designed to protect, promote, and improve the health and well-being of students and staff, thus improving a student's ability to learn. It includes, but is not limited to, comprehensive school health education; school health services; a healthy school environment; school counseling; psychological and social services; physical education; school nutrition services; family and community involvement in school health; and school-site health promotion for staff.

Determinants of Health

Biological, environmental, behavioral, organizational, political, and social factors that contribute to the health status of individuals, groups, and communities.

Evidence-Based Health Education

The systematic selection, implementation, and evaluation of strategies, programs, and policies, with evidence from the scientific literature that they have demonstrated effectiveness in accomplishing intended outcomes.

Formative Assessment

"Ongoing assessment providing data to guide instruction and improve performance." Carr, J. F., and D. E. Harris. 2001. *Succeeding with Standards: Linking Curriculum, Assessment, and Action Planning.* Alexandria, VA: Association for Supervision and Curriculum Development.

Health Advocacy

The processes by which the actions of individuals or groups attempt to bring about social and organizational change on behalf of the particular health goal, program, interest, or population.

Health Education

Any combination of planned learning experiences based on sound theories that provide individuals, groups, and communities the opportunity to acquire information and the skills needed to make quality health decisions.

Health Education Field

A practice that uses multidisciplinary theories and behavioral and organizational change principles to plan, implement, and evaluate interventions that enable individuals, groups and communities to achieve personal, environmental, and social health.

Health Educator

A professionally prepared individual who serves in a variety of roles and is specifically trained to use appropriate educational strategies and methods to facilitate the development of policies, procedures, interventions, and systems conducive to the health of individuals, groups, and communities to achieve personal, environmental, and social health.

Health Information

The content of communications derived from credible sources related to individual, group, and community health issues and concerns.

Health Literacy

The capacity of an individual to obtain, interpret, and understand basic health information and services and the competence to use such information and services in ways that are health enhancing.

Health Outcome

Measurable change in or reinforcement of factors related to health status or quality of life attributable to a series of events, whether planned or unplanned.

Health Promotion

Any planned combination of educational, political, environmental, regulatory, or organizational mechanisms that support actions and conditions of living conducive to the health of individuals, groups, and communities.

Healthy Lifestyle

Patterns of behavior that maximize one's quality of life and decrease one's susceptibility to negative health outcomes.

High-Stakes Tests

"Tests used to determine which individual students get rewards, honors, or sanctions. Low-stakes tests are used primarily to improve student learning. Tests with high stakes attached include college entrance examinations and tests students must pass to be promoted to the next grade. Tests affecting the status of schools, such as those on which a given percentage of students must receive a passing grade, are also considered high stakes." (Association for Supervision and Curriculum Development)

Norm-Referenced Assessment

"An assessment where student performance or performances are compared to [those of] a larger group. Usually the larger group or 'norm group' is a national sample representing a wide and diverse cross section of students. Students, schools, districts, and even states are compared or rank-ordered in relation to the norm group. The purpose of a norm-referenced assessment is usually to sort students and not to measure achievement toward some criterion of performance." (National Center for Research on Evaluation, Standards, and Student Testing, 1999)

Norm-Referenced Tests

"Standardized tests designed to measure how a student's performance compares with that of other students. Most standardized achievement tests are norm-referenced, meaning that a student's performance is compared to the performances of students in a norming group. Scores on norm-referenced tests are often reported in terms of grade-level equivalencies or percentiles derived from the scores of the original students." (Association for Supervision and Curriculum Development)

Observation Scales

"Observation scales define specific performances (desired skills and behaviors) of students and also may identify a developmental range of student behavior that moves toward criterion performance. Teachers are trained to systematically observe students in multiple environments to evaluate performance. Observation scales are useful in evaluating student progress toward a standard and often encourage evaluation based on a holistic picture of the student as a learner." (North Central Regional Educational Laboratory)

Performance Assessment

"A form of assessment designed to assess what students know" or should be able to do "through their ability to perform certain tasks. For example, demonstrating how to refuse pressure to use tobacco, using the Internet to access valid health information about alcohol and other drugs, writing a letter to advocate for safe spaces and facilities for physical activities, or creating a plan to monitor goals related to healthy eating." (Adapted from Association for Supervision and Curriculum Development)

Performance Task

"Activities, exercises, or problems that require students to show what they can do. Some performance tasks are intended to assess a skill. Others are designed to have students demonstrate their understanding by applying knowledge . . ." (Association for Supervision and Curriculum Development)

Portfolio

"A collection of student work chosen to exemplify and document a student's learning progress over time." (Association for Supervision and Curriculum Development)

Portfolio Assessment

"A portfolio is a collection of work, usually drawn from students' classroom work. A portfolio becomes a portfolio assessment when (1) the assessment purpose is defined; (2) criteria or methods are made clear for determining what is put into the portfolio, by whom, and when; and (3) criteria for assessing either the collection or individual pieces of work are identified and used to make judgments about performance. Portfolios can be designed to assess student progress, effort, and/or achievement, and to encourage students to reflect on their learning." (National Center for Research on Evaluation, Standards, and Student Testing, 1999)

Prevention

Actions and interventions designed to identify risks and reduce susceptibility or exposure to health threats prior to disease onset (primary prevention), detect and treat disease in early stages to prevent progress or recurrence (secondary prevention), and alleviate the effects of disease and injury (tertiary prevention).

Reliability

"The degree to which the results of an assessment are dependable and consistently measure particular student knowledge and/or skills. Reliability is an indication of the consistency of scores across raters, over time, or across different tasks or items that measure the same thing. Thus, reliability may be expressed as (a) the relationship between test items intended to measure the same skill or knowledge (item reliability), (b) the relationship between two administrations of the same test to the same student or students (test/retest reliability), or (c) the degree of agreement between two or more raters (rater reliability). An unreliable assessment cannot be valid." (National Center for Research on Evaluation, Standards, and Student Testing, 1999)

Risk Reduction

Actions that can successfully decrease the probability that individuals, groups, or communities will experience disease or debilitating health conditions.

Rubric

"A set of guidelines for scoring student work. A typical rubric states the assessment criteria, contains a scale and helps educators rate student work according to the scale." Council of Chief State School Officers. 1997. *Assessing Health Literacy: A Guide to Portfolios. Washington, DC: Council of Chief State School Officers,* p. 97. See also "Analytical Rubric" and "Holistic Rubric."

Self-Efficacy

"Beliefs in one's capabilities to organize and execute a course of action required to produce given attainments." Bandura, A. 1997. *Self-Efficacy: The Exercise of Control.* New York: W. H. Freemand and Co., p. 3.

School Health Coordinator

A certificated or licensed professional at the state, district, or school level who is responsible for managing, coordinating, implementing, and evaluating all school health policies, activities, and resources.

Skill Cues

The elements of skills that the students should be able to demonstrate as a result of instruction. The skill cues for advocacy, for example, include "takes a clear, health-enhancing stand/position; supports the position with relevant information; shows awareness of audience; encourages others to make healthful choices; demonstrates passion/conviction."

Standards-Based Assessment

"Criterion-referenced assessment in which the criteria are taken directly from standards." (Carr and Harris, 2001, p. 185)

Standards-Based Education

"Teaching directed toward student mastery of defined standards. Now that nearly all states have adopted curriculum standards, teachers are expected to teach in such a way that students achieve the standards. Experts say this means that teachers must have a clear idea what each standard means, including how it can and will be assessed, and that teachers should monitor individual student achievement of each important standard." (Association for Supervision and Curriculum Development)

Summative Assessment

"A snapshot of student performance at a given time, judged according to pre-established standards and criteria. Summative assessment typically leads to a status report on success or degree of proficiency." (Carr and Harris, 2001, p. 186)

Summative Test
"A test given to evaluate what students have learned. The term is used to distinguish such tests from formative tests, which are used primarily to diagnose what students have learned in order to plan further instruction." (Association for Supervision and Curriculum Development)

Validity
"The extent to which an assessment measures what it is supposed to measure and the extent to which inferences and actions made on the basis of test scores are appropriate and accurate." (National Center for Research on Evaluation, Standards, and Student Testing, 1999)

Wellness
An approach to health that focuses on balancing the many aspects or dimensions of a person's life through increasing the adoption of health-enhancing conditions and behaviors, rather than attempting to minimize conditions of illness.

Notes

Notes

Notes

Notes

Notes

Notes

Notes

Notes

NATIONAL
HEALTH
EDUCATION
STANDARDS

National Health Education Standards

SECOND EDITION

ACHIEVING EXCELLENCE

Available Now in 3 Convenient Formats!

1 Printed book
$29.95 USD
ACS Product Code #**2027.27**
ISBN 13: 978-0-944235-73-7

2 CD-ROM
$19.95 USD
ACS Product Code #**2027.24**
ISBN 13: 978-0-944235-83-6

3 Downloadable PDF
(online prepayment only)
$9.95 USD
ACS Product Code #**2027.25**
ISBN 13: 978-0-944235-84-3

How to Order Individual Copies

Order all of these products directly from the American Cancer Society.
Call us toll free 1.800.ACS.2345 or shop online at **www.cancer.org/NHES**
All major credit cards accepted.

How to Order Bulk Quantities and/or Send Purchase Orders

Send POs for any quantity of the **printed book and/or CD-ROM** to us by fax (404.325.9341) or by email (trade.sales@cancer.org).

Or use the handy paper ORDER FORM on next page.

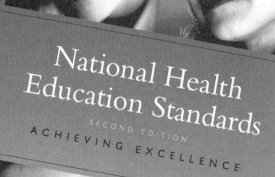

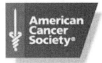

Order Your Copies Today!
Fax to: **404.325.9341**
Email to: **trade.sales@cancer.org**

National Health Education Standards
SECOND EDITION
ACHIEVING EXCELLENCE

Developed by the Joint Committee on National Health Education Standards

Supported by the American Cancer Society, the Joint Committee membership and selected experts in the field of health education conducted a 10-year review and revision of the 1995 National Health Education Standards. Collaborative partners included the American Association for Health Education, the American School Health Association, the American Public Health Association, and the Society of State Directors of Health, Physical Education and Recreation.

PO #: _____ Date: _____

FORM OF PAYMENT

☐ Purchase order   ☐ Check #_____   ☐ Visa   ☐ Master Card   ☐ American Express

Credit card # _____ *Expiration date* _____

Name on card _____

Authorized signature _____

☐ I wish to receive notification of other ACS books. My email address: _____

BILLING AND SHIPPING INFORMATION

Bill to: **Ship to ★via** ☐ UPS Ground   ☐ Fed Ex

Name   Name

Company   Company

Street address   Street address (no P.O.boxes)

Suite/Floor   Suite/Floor

City/State/Zip   City/State/Zip

Qty	Product/Format	ACS Prod Code	ISBN-13	List	Total
_____	**NHES Printed Book**	# 2027.27	978-0-944235-73-7	$29.95	_____
_____	**NHES CD-ROM**	# 2027.24	978-0-944235-83-6	$19.95	_____

Subtotal $_____

Organization's Sales Tax Exemption Certificate #_____

Georgia residents will be charged applicable sales tax.

SHIPPING CHARGE WILL BE APPLIED TO ALL INVOICED ORDERS.

All products will ship via UPS Ground, unless another delivery method is specified and/or customer's account number is provided **at the time the order is placed.**